10   GIFORD (DRAFTED)

100   CUTAWAY THROAT WOUND

128-9   BACK BRACE — NURSES & GREER —ELASTIC 6"WIDE

163   GOOD DESCRIPTION OF SHOOTING ABILITIES

190   BARK BRACE   CANVAS & METAL   ?

236   "WHAT HAPPENED TO BODY BRACE AND ACE BANDAGE"

Medicolegal Investigation
of the
President John F. Kennedy Murder

Medicolegal Investigation
of the
President John F. Kennedy Murder

By

CHARLES G. WILBER, Ph.D.

Fellow, American Academy of Forensic Sciences
Deputy Coroner, Larimer County, Colorado
Director, Forensic Science Laboratory
Colorado State University
Fort Collins, Colorado

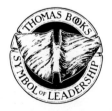

CHARLES C THOMAS • **PUBLISHER**
Springfield • Illinois • U.S.A.

Published and Distributed Throughout the World by
CHARLES C THOMAS • PUBLISHER
Bannerstone House
301-327 East Lawrence Avenue, Springfield, Illinois, U.S.A.

© *1978, by* CHARLES C THOMAS • PUBLISHER

ISBN 0-398-03679-9

Library of Congress Catalog Card Number: 77-8567

Printed in the United States of America
OO-2

Library of Congress Cataloging in Publication Data

Wilber, Charles Grady, 1916-
　　Medicolegal investigation of the President John F.
　　Kennedy murder.

　　Bibliography: p.
　　Includes index.
　　1. Kennedy, John Fitzgerald, Pres. U. S., 1917-
1963--Assassination.　2. Kennedy, John Fitzgerald,
Pres. U. S., 1917-1963--Autopsy.　3. Autopsy.
4. Gunshot wounds.　I. Title.
E842.9.W466　　　614'.19　　　77-8567
ISBN 0-398-03679-9

PREFACE

THE murder of President John F. Kennedy was an event in the history of the United States that left deep and lasting wounds in the body politic and social structure. Kennedy, a relatively young man as American presidents go, had not accomplished much as chief executive; his decisions were not particularly remarkable or effective. His great genius was that he had captured the emotions and the imagination of the common people; he had rekindled in Americans a pride that said we could accomplish anything to which we put our collective mind and resources.

It is also important to recall that he was a Catholic. His election forever obliterated the silly and despicable prejudice that a Catholic president would turn the nation over to the Vatican State. Now it no longer matters whether a Catholic is elected to or even runs for president. When such can be said also for Jews, blacks, women, and other groups artifically pigeonholed in American society, then this nation can be said to have reached a mature status.

The murder itself was carried out in plain view of thousands of people. Radio announcers were reporting; television cameras were presumably grinding; photographers of all sorts — amateur, professional, still, and motion picture — were exposing their films as the event took place. Police at the local level and federal police were thronged around the murder area. Despite this assemblage of information-gathering and recording sources, the murder of John F. Kennedy is still, in the minds of most people in the United States and indeed of the world, an unresolved problem obscured by deceit, ineptitude, and official wrongheadedness.

A commission was appointed by President Lyndon Johnson to wring out, from *all* the evidence, the truth of what occurred.

The production of that Commission was and is a disaster. For the first time, as a consequence of the Commission's official report, the American people began to be aware that their government used the lie, cover-up, double-talk, and secrecy as tools of governing.* The end result of the latter 1970s has been a growing cynicism about the American system and the American dream. Repair of this unfortunate state of affairs must begin with a reevaluation of the entire complex situation of the Kennedy murder.

This book concerns itself only with the medicolegal aspects of the John F. Kennedy assassination. It is not intended to explore the details of international relations, federal police, or spies in the domestic and foreign scene. The book is primarily based on an evaluation of the medicolegal facts as available by a forensic scientist and practicing death investigator.

To my mind, there are such great inconsistencies in the summary Report published by the Warren Commission, as its official conclusion, and the twenty-six volumes of evidence and exhibits collected by the Commission and published by the Government Printing Office that a thorough, impartial, and reliable (credible?) reinvestigation is mandatory.

The inconsistencies are well illustrated by the strange medicolegal conclusions of the Commission that are so frequently at variance with the professional testimony of physicians and other experts.

From the first I was seriously disturbed by the autopsy report and the handling of physical evidence in the case. Later I read the responses of allegedly thoughtful and reliable persons to critical analyses of the Warren Commission findings. The invective, the *argumentum ad hominem,* and the strident responses of the defenders of the Report led me to the view that the Report was not very strong and that its defenders were

---

*This incipient awareness was to become full-blown as a result of the action of subsequent "blue ribbon" commissions that purported to study such matters as pornography, social violence, criminal justice, marijuana, and other matters of national concern. Confidence in and respect for the central government has eroded to an alarming degree.

emotionally in a panic. It, therefore, seemed appropriate to go through the chaotically organized twenty-six volumes of Hearing and Exhibits to ascertain what information was actually collected by the Commission. The exercise was revealing but disturbing. The Report was apparently written with preconceived ideas plugged in. The Hearings and Exhibits were used when the prewritten Report found the data supportive; they were ignored or suppressed when no support (or even contradiction) was given the prewritten script.

In addition to the inadequacies and distortions of the officially published volumes, there are the grave questions created by the governmental handling of the mass of Commission documents that were not published and are presumably on file in the National Archives. These files include crucial material of a medicolegal nature; the suppression (or even possible destruction) of this material suggests that something needs to be kept secret.

As the secret Kennedy murder materials in the National Archives collection have leaked out in bits and pieces, it becomes clear that the FBI resorted to lies in response to queries about certain evidence, the Warren Commission itself probably subscribed knowingly to lies, and various federal agencies have, with a high degree of probability, been guilty of destroying materials relevant to the case.

An Example of Suppressed Information

Unexpected news releases by government agencies from time to time try the faith of Americans in the integrity of the Warren Commission as a group and as individuals. For example, the following news release was carried on national radio and television services on 13 November 1976.

A memorandum from late FBI Director, J. Edgar Hoover, has recently come to light. In that document, Lee Harvey Oswald is said to have told Fidel Castro that he, Oswald, planned to murder President John F. Kennedy. A highly reliable source is said to have revealed the matter to Hoover after being himself told of it by Castro. This memorandum, if true, suggests that Castro or his henchmen were involved in Kennedy's murder in retaliation for CIA attempts to kill Castro.

Reportedly, shortly after Oswald told Castro of his plans, he (Oswald) got a job at the Texas Book Depository Building. Detailed plans of the precise route that the presidential cavalcade would take through Dallas were presumably not firm until long after that time. Oswald's preknowledge of just what building would be ideal for his sniper attempt even before the parade route was allegedly selected is remarkable to say the least, especially for a nonentity working alone and with no help from anyone but himself.

Find a Better Answer

In response to critics of the conclusions published by the Warren Commission, many of its defenders have asserted that unless the critic comes up with a better answer and points the finger of guilt at a specific person other than Oswald (with all the necessary evidence), then the criticism is invalid and is the product of a warped mind or of a sensation seeker.

Such a contention is intellectually dishonest; those who take that pose know that it is dishonest.

The iron curtain of secrecy that has been drawn between the available documents and materials in the total file connected with the Kennedy murder and competent scholars who wish to study the record makes it impossible to move ahead until the rules are changed and the searchlight of scholarship is allowed to play over every note, minute, and speck of dust accumulated as part of the record. The record includes files and other materials squirreled away in obscure places other than the National Archives.

Because of the "stacked deck," as it were, the present book is based heavily on the public record made available in the public domain. When that material is put together, especially the medicolegal parts, it becomes obvious that the conclusions of the Warren Commission as published in the official Report are remarkably unsupported by the very evidence put into the

Record by the Commission staff.

A number of books are available to the ordinary reader who wishes to follow up certain details of the murder of John F. Kennedy. A basic volume to any study of the assassination is the Report of the President's Commission on the Assassination of President Kennedy (1964). It is available from the Government Printing Office and can be examined in most public libraries. The Rockefeller *Report to the President by the Commission on CIA Activities within the United States* (1975) is also available. It must be read with extreme caution because, in general, it is not honest, complete, forthright, or reliable. In essence the report on the CIA relied on the CIA to investigate itself.

One of the earliest and most scholarly of the studies on the murder of President Kennedy was produced by Sylvia Meagher (1967); it has been recently republished in paperback form by Random House (1976). It is recommended to all persons who have a serious interest in the assassination. Meagher (1966) also created a subject index to the jumble of Hearings and Exhibits put together by the Commission into twenty-six volumes as supporting material for the Report. The index is of great value to students of the assassination; unfortunately it has been out of print for some time.

Scott, Hoch, and Stetler (1976) have put together a useful anthology of writings about the John F. Kennedy assassination. One of the earliest books to call attention to questionable aspects of the Warren Commission conclusions was *Rush to Judgement* by Lane (1966); it has come out more recently in paperback form. Bishop wrote a popular account of the shooting in 1968; a paperback edition was available in 1973. The book is completely supportive of the Warren Commission findings. An anthology of writings about the murder has been put together by Blumenthal and Yazijian (1976).

A book that deserves serious attention has been written by Anson (1975). The author is a seasoned newsman; he includes in his work a detailed analysis of the color motion picture sequence of the shooting as well as an evaluation of the changing physical measurements of Oswald.

Other books are also available for those who have access to a good book store: Model and Groden (1976), Garrison (1970), Weisberg (1965), Fox (1965), Noyes (1973).

This listing does not pretend to be all-inclusive. It does give the reader a selection of books available for study. No attempt has been made to include personally published books or pamphlets dealing with the subject. Many of these contain valuable information and ideas. However, they are difficult to come by; the average reader has neither the time nor the patience to track them down.

Numerous serial articles have been written about the assassination; they have appeared in a variety of publications from *Playboy* to the *Journal of Forensic Sciences*. Only those that are actually used as a reference in this book are listed in the literature cited.

A Thought to Ponder

It is ironic that presumably sophisticated government bureaucrats and politicians do not understand one of the elementary facts of living: A lie begets further lies. A simple, possibly harmless, series of lies incorporated in the Warren Commission Report has required further lies to cover up the original lies. The result is a chain reaction of one lie built upon another in order continuously to cover up the track of prevarication. The average citizen understands this fact of living. How government bureaucrats seem to be unaware of this fact suggests that something is wrong with our choosing of governmental leaders. Something is wrong with our system of education that permits individuals of this sort to rise to high levels of public responsibility without having developed a keen awareness of the devastating results of lying as an official policy. To argue that the end result was so important that it justified these lies is reprehensible, naive, and counterproductive. No lie can ever be justified in terms of the end result. For, in the long run, an official lie begins a chain of further lies so that when the truth finally surfaces, there is revealed a stinking morass of interlocking lies that have caused long-term, if not permanent, damage to the government subscribing to such a procedure and to the people afflicted with such a government.

There is little doubt that something in the assassination record is unsavory. Bureaucratic idiocy cannot explain the persistent refusal by all levels of the federal government to share with the public the records of the Kennedy murder. The collusion of the courts in this disgraceful secrecy is of grave concern to all thoughtful citizens.

Appeals to national security, "good taste," sensitivity, and the like are dishonest and insulting; they reveal a deep-seated contempt for citizens on the part of too many federal officials.

Collusion?

The various federal courts have cooperated with the bureaucrats of the central government to keep a barrier of secrecy (domestic curtain of iron?) between the total records of the Warren Commission and the people of this nation.

Among the more deceitful rulings issued by the United States Supreme Court was one dated 13 May 1974 to the effect that the Freedom of Information Act does not force the Department of Justice to open for public inspection spectrographic reports made on the fragments of bullets allegedly used in the murder of late President John F. Kennedy (Facts on File, 1974).

Collusion between the administrative and the judicial branches of the central government to hide information of grave public interest seems obvious.

At the end of this book there will be a series of conclusions based on the evidence that is available; the conclusions are those of the author, who is a forensic biologist and an active member of the coroner's office. This experience as a coroner's deputy, as well as active research in the subject of wound ballistics, will obviously aid in the formulation of the conclusions.

In the past, enthusiastic defenders of the Commission and its Report have done little to clarify issues; they certainly have not helped to get hidden data into the light of day.

The usual tactics in the past used against adverse critics of the Report or of the Commission operations fall under the general umbrella of *argumentum ad hominem.* This device was known to the ancient world; it has been despised by all honest men since then as a shameful ploy used to subvert the truth.

Essentially the device is to ignore the argument or issue and to attack the proponent. The oponent must be degraded; his morals and integrity must be defamed; hidden evils in his character and base motives for his thesis must be whispered, but never must the thesis itself be analyzed in an objective manner. Thus, if the critic has clay feet, his thesis must be wrong. This logical fallacy has been the usual one inflicted on those who have criticized the Report.

It is hoped that with the passage of time this sort of anti-intellectual response will have died away. The problem is too important for our country and for the world at large to have it besmirched by the injection of cheap debate tricks into a sincere and grave evaluation.

Reviews and rejoinders based on intellectual considerations will be studied with interest in a positive way. Scurrilous comments and evaluations based on the *argumentum ad hominem* fallacy will be given the disposition they earn — a total disregard of their existence.

A peculiar fact emerges from the unpublished material in the National Archives files (Commission Document No. 5, p. 400). Lee Harvey Oswald was never charged or arraigned in connection with the death of President John F. Kennedy. Oswald himself asserted as much when questioned by newsmen. Did Chief Curry of the Dallas police perjure himself when he claimed to be present at the time Oswald was arraigned for killing President Kennedy? Did other police officers commit perjury when they supported, under oath, Curry's testimony?

Oswald was charged only with the murder of Dallas police officer Tippit according to unpublished records of the Warren Commission.*

---

*According to the Report (p. 198), shortly after 1:30 a.m. Oswald was brought to the identification bureau on the fourth floor and arraigned before Justice of the Peace Johnston, that time for the murder of President Kennedy (Hearings, vol. 4, pp. 155, 221; Commission Exhibit No. 2003, p. 104; Hearings, vol. 15, pp. 507-508). The Report further stated (p. 200) that on Friday afternoon "about 5 hours later (than what?), he

→

It is of great interest that Chief Justice Warren himself admitted that the whole truth of the matter may never be known in our lifetimes. Such admission is incredible but undisputed.

A book of this sort requires much help. With gratitude I wish to thank Sally Carson of New York City for her role as unpaid research assistant, my wife, Clare M. Wilber, who carried out the reading of proof, and the following members of the office staff, Department of Zoology and Entomology, Colorado State University, for heroic efforts in typing the final drafts of the chapters: Barbara Alldredge, Janelle Q. Simon, Sharon Sonday, and Susan Berry.

Finally, I thank the various audiences before whom I tried out portions of this book for their critical questioning and their encouragement to "make a book of it."

Charles G. Wilber, Ph.D.

---

was arraigned for the Tippit murder and within an additional 6 1/2 hours he was arraigned for the murder of President Kennedy." By Friday midnight, the Report admits (p. 201) that "at this time Oswald had been arraigned only for the murder of Patrolman Tippit. . . ." It is also apparent from the record that at no time did Oswald *de facto* have legal counsel.

CONTENTS

Medicolegal Investigation
of the
President John F. Kennedy Murder

CHAPTER 1

INTRODUCTION

O N Friday 22 November 1963 President John F. Kennedy was gunned down while participating in a motorcade through the streets of Dallas, Texas. Shortly after the killing, President Lyndon Johnson appointed a President's Commission to investigate the assassination of President John F. Kennedy. As soon as the report of the Commission had been issued, it generated a worldwide storm of protest and disbelief. That rejection of the Report as a document worthy of belief has been so widespread that today eight out of ten Americans discard the conclusions of the Report as having any validity.*

What went wrong? Why is there such virtually universal repudiation of the Commission and its work? Are most of the people of the world perverse and blind to the facts of history, or is there objective reason for rejecting the Report?

A detailed examination of the basic Report and the twenty-six volumes of Hearings and Exhibits discloses an amazing pattern of strange coincidences and questionable behavior that conspire to vitiate the arguments leading to the official conclusions of the Commission.

The official version of what happened that day in Dallas is bloated with irrelevances and is skeletonized in many critical parts.

Significant forensic science evidence included in the Hearings and Exhibits supports the contention that more than one individual was involved in the actual shooting of the President in Dallas. The Warren Commission opted to pick and choose

---

*Students of history may never unearth all of what actually happened on 22 November 1963 in Dallas. Why, for example, were federal police not covering the roofs of buildings that commanded a view of the murder site? A possible simple but logical answer may be buried in the records of a federal operating agency and may in essence be unavailable to scholars. Nevertheless, "Historians must be eternal skeptics of evidence whose original cannot be probed" (Wrone, 1972). Too much of the so-called medical evidence in the John F. Kennedy murder case falls into that category.

3

evidence that supported the single, unaided assassin postulate.

Official secrecy that has stubbornly persisted even in the face of laws passed specifically to break that secrecy, the hiding of items material to the investigation and the possible destruction or mutilation of critical physical evidence have contrived to cast doubt even on the laudable parts of the Commission Report.

What is the official version of the death of John F. Kennedy?

First of all, the Commission concluded that the President was killed by a lone assassin named Lee Harvey Oswald who had no confederates, discussed the matter with no one, and received no support or aid in any form from another person or persons. His motives were obscure but the Commission implied that he was "insane." The Commission emphasized as a key point that no "conspiracy" was involved.

However, even a cursory reading of the official Report reveals language that hedges at crucial points in the document. There is a skilled use of English which serves well to obscure the fact that the Commission admits uncertainty with respect to the number of shots that were actually fired in Dallas on that fateful day. Uncertainty is evident with respect to the sequence of shots and just how Governor Connally was wounded. The origin of the various shots is also a matter of quandry.

Central to the Commission's conclusions is the strange theory of the "single bullet" that is said to have passed through the body of President Kennedy from back to front (causing minor wounds), passed through Governor Connally, smashing the rib and a wrist, and leaving a trail of metal particles in the Governor's body, and then emerged in a virtually pristine state except for rifling marks engraved on its sides, but with no deformation of any degree.

Much concern surrounds the one bullet theory, because from various sources it is evident that the President and Connally were wounded within 1.5 seconds of one another. The rifle alleged to have been used in the murder could not have been fired that rapidly at a moving target even by skilled riflemen. The Commission was faced with the dilemma: Either one bullet caused the nonfatal wounds in Kennedy and Connally or two rifles fired by separate shooters had to be involved. At the urging of Arlen Specter, a young assistant district attorney from Philadelphia, the Commission opted for the one bullet theory.

The story of the one bullet that is concluded to have gone through both the President and the Governor is so strange that it contributes much to the disbelief aroused by the Report. The bullet, after wounding two men and smashing two bones in one of them, is said to have fallen out of a bone-deep thigh wound in Governor Connally. It then was found under the pad on a stretcher near an elevator door in a remote part of Parkland Hospital by a janitor. Whether Kennedy or Connally ever occupied the stretcher in question is doubtful. The finder of the bullet refused to swear who occupied the stretcher. Several hospital employees swear that the cart on which the bullet was found had been used for a little boy who was brought in by his mother because of a severely bleeding accidental wound.

The bullet is a 6.5 mm Mannlicher-Carcano slug. It has a lead core covered with a copper jacket, except for the base of the bullet, which has lead exposed. Rifling marks engraved on the sides of the copper jacket are said by the FBI to prove that the bullet was fired from the alleged murder weapon. The nose is undeformed. The weight of the discovered bullet is 158.6 grains; the average weight of bullets from unfired cartridges of that same kind is 161 grains.

The bullet looks very much like those that have been fired into a long tube filled with cotton waste so that the slug can be recovered for ballistic studies — undeformed but with the rifling marks intact.

A basic question, unanswered and probably unanswerable, keeps arising. "How could a bullet cause so much bone damage and yet be absolutely undeformed?" (Wilber, 1977).

The Commission had a government agency at Edgewood Arsenal in Maryland run tests to substantiate the one bullet theory. The tests and results have not been completely revealed. What results are known fail to support the one bullet theory.

Some Considerations on the Assassination of President Kennedy

Among the many factors which have raised questions in the

minds of forensic scientists concerning the formal Report of the Hearings before the President's Commission on the Assassination of President Kennedy (1964) are some of the peculiarities of the Hearing itself. Presumably, the Chief Justice of the Supreme Court of the United States presided at these hearings. Consequently, one would anticipate that all the legal nuances and technicalities written into our laws would be respected in these hearings.

Quite the contrary obtained, however. For example, on page 349 of volume 2 of the Commission Hearings, Commander Humes, who conducted the autopsy on the President's remains, began his testimony with what can be considered a remarkable statement. He said, "When apprised of the necessity for our appearance before this Commission, we did not know whether or not the photographs, which we had made, would be available to the Commission." This situation occurred in the later part of the twentieth century. The statement was describing probably the most important medicolegal autopsy of the twentieth century. Incredible as it is, the basic data from the autopsy were not available to the *one key person* who was testifying nor to the Commission that was pretending to investigate the assassination. There is no conceivable excuse that could possibly justify such a situation.

Instead of presenting photographs made at the autopsy and x-rays also taken during the course of the autopsy, a procedure that would have been routine in any other kind of investigation, an enlisted medical corps sailor was assigned to produce what were called by Commander Humes "schematic drawings." These schematics were based on oral instructions from Commander Humes and several of his associates. Oral descriptions only were available to the sailor who was supposed to draw a meaningful sketch of the wounds including size, location, and the like.

The further exchange between Arlen Specter (a lawyer for the Commission) and Doctor Humes about photographs as routine devices at autopsies is informative. Mr. Specter asked Doctor Humes, "Would it be helpful to the artist, in redefining the drawings if that should be necessary, to have available to him photographs or X-rays of the President?"

This question was either mischievous or uninformed. Any ordinary citizen in his right mind would know that a photograph of a wound is essential to give precise location, shape, etc. No artist's drawing, no matter how precise and exact, can reflect the nature of a wound.

Commander Humes answered, "If it were necessary to have them absolutely true to scale. I think it would be virtually impossible for him to do this without the photographs." Specter was obviously trying to becloud the whole issue when he followed up this discussion with another question, "And what is the reason for the necessity for having photographs?"

I wonder how many ordinary citizens with no legal or medical training there are who would have any doubts about the desirability and indeed the necessity for having photographs if one wants to see precisely the nature of a wound. Commander Humes tried to answer the question as best he could. He said, "I think that it is most difficult to transmit into physical measurements the — by word the — exact situation as it would seem to the naked eye. The photographs were — there is no problem of scale there because the wounds, if they are changed in size or changed in size and proportion to the structures of the body, etc., when we attempt to give a description of these findings, it is the bony prominences, I cannot, which we used as points of references, I cannot transmit completely to the illustrator where they were situated." In spite of the fact that this answer is a transcript of an oral response to a silly question, it is clear that Commander Humes was trying to point out that there is no way by using words alone to impart to an illustrator the exact size, shape, relationships, etc. of wounds so that they can be located in a drawing with any degree of precision.

Mr. Specter continued along this line and asked another mischievous question (certainly the question makes no sense when asked by a lawyer who knows better). He said, "Is the taking of photographs and X-rays routine or is this something out of the ordinary?" Commander Humes again patiently answered, "No sir; this is quite routine in cases of this sort of violent death in our training period. In the field of forensic pathology we have found that the photographs and X-rays are of most value, the X-rays, particularly in finding missiles which have a way of going in different directions sometimes, and particularly as documentary evidence these are considered invaluable in the field of forensic pathology."

Clearly Doctor Humes, who was certified as an anatomical and clinical pathologist, recognized without equivocation that photographs and x-rays provide documentary evidence that is *invaluable* in the field for forensic pathology. One wonders how much stronger the answer could have been made to break through the collective stupidity of the Commission in refusing to demand that photographs and x-rays be made available so that the individual testifying could clarify with confidence the exact condition of the wounds.

Armed Forces regulations demand that sketches and photographs that are made be included as integral parts of the autopsy report.

A Bungled Autopsy

A series of schematics based on remembrances of the autopsy pathologists and transmitted orally to a naval enlisted man was used as the basis for critical testimony by the pathologists concerning the nature of the wounds inflicted on the President. The enlisted artist was asked to produce drawings to be used in court without having any direct access to photographs or x-rays of the body. Neither had the enlisted artist been at the autopsy to see the wounds firsthand. His artistic creations are hearsay evidence of the classical type; but the Commission forced the situation and accepted the charts and the testimony on the charts, a strange kind of behavior for the Chief Justice of the United States Supreme Court to show. It is obvious then that the basic medicolegal data accepted by the Warren Commission is tainted and open to grave question.

It is no wonder that grave questions of fact arise in the minds of serious scholars faced with the unexplainable disregard of primary autopsy evidence on the part of the investigating Commission. The end result of deleting pictures and x-rays from the autopsy report and the obvious "editing" of the text of the report itself leaves one faced with a bungled autopsy in the record.

A favorite aphorism of Lacassagne, one of the founders of modern forensic science follows: "A bungled autopsy cannot be revised" (Thorwald, 1965). Accumulated experience over a century since then has confirmed Lacassagne's warning.

The aphorism suggests that too much must not be expected from any reinvestigation of the John F. Kennedy postmortem examination. The autopsy at Bethesda Naval Hospital was admittedly bungled, and bungled badly. Can it be revised so as to reveal the truth, the whole truth, and nothing but the truth?

The prospects for ever uncovering the complete and true story of the murder of John F. Kennedy are dim. The work of destroying the impact of the autopsy on the investigation of the case has been carried out only too well.

Nevertheless, it is important that what medicolegal data are still available be critically reevaluated in order to provide the historical record with a more nearly competent study of one of the major events of the twentieth century.

The Evidence

The Warren Commission stoutly maintained that all the relevant and meaningful evidence connected with the murder of President John F. Kennedy was included, without equivocation, in the official Report and supporting documents. Every administration since then has repeated the claim and has denied that there is justification for reopening the investigation or probing into the mounds of documentation buried in the National Archives until the year 2039 A.D.

All these sources contend that the published evidence supports, with no possibility of contradiction, the formal conclusions of the Warren Commission.*

---

*The editing and the reproduction of photographs in the Exhibit volumes of the Commission publication are bewilderingly below the usual high quality that one

Many apologists for the validity, without question, of the Warren Report agree in this contention.

The latest official paper published in support of the Warren Commission Report is the Report to the President by the Commission on CIA Activities Within the United States. It supports every comma and period in the Warren Commission Report (Rockefeller, 1975).

Gerald Ford, while still in the House of Representatives, served as a member of the Warren Commission. He later wrote a book to justify the conclusions of the Commission. On 3 April 1975 there was an interesting give-and-take between reporters and Ford, who was then an appointed president of the United States. Ford was asked whether he still had confidence in the Commission's conclusions after the many public showings of the Zapruder film (Scott, Hoch, and Stetler, 1976). Ford replied, "I think you'd have to read very carefully what the Warren Commission said, and I as a member of the Warren Commissions helped to participate in the drafting of the language." He also admitted that the Commission pointed to Oswald as the murderer. Then he added, "We said that the commission had found no evidence of a conspiracy, foreign or domestic. *Those words were very carefully drafted ... "* (emphasis added).

What is meant by that last sentence? One interpretation is ominous; the Commission really said nothing. Could it be that the rejection of autopsy evidence and other data was planned so that the carefully worded "no conspiracy" conclusion was on the surface true, but only because of culpable ignorance on the part of the Commission?

A later phrase suggests that perhaps this question has an affirmative answer. Ford said, "But the commission was right when it made its determination and it was accurate at least to this point and I want to reemphasize that as to the evidence

---

expects from the Government Printing Office. For example, Commission Exhibit Numbers 840, 842, and 843 are fragments of presumed bullets pertinent to the Kennedy murder case. The lighting in the pictures is flat; the texture of the fragments is virtually nonexistent. Moreover, none of the pictures shows a reference line; the actual size of the fragments thus cannot be estimated, a fact that makes the pictures comparatively useless (Hearings, vol. 17, pp. 840, 841).

that we saw." This is a strange disclaimer. Did the Commission see only what it wanted to see or what the staff wanted it to see?

In the face of these weighty confirmations of the official Report on John F. Kennedy's murder, it is not inappropriate to use the basic medicolegal data published by the Commission as a foundation for a critique of the conclusions of the Commission. Since, by the Commission's own declaration defended vigorously by all federal administrations since then and by individual members of the Commission and its staff, every scrap of pertinent medicolegal evidence has been included in the published Report, it is fair to base a medicolegal reevaluation of the conclusions on what basic data have been published in the Report.

On the basis of official statements repeated again and again, it is fair to assume that no new revelations or evidence can come from official sources to confuse and confound such a new evaluation. Specifically, the official and emphatic contention has been that no relevant unpublished data are in the unpublished files of the Commission.

It is long overdue that the medicolegal data be evaluated by a professional forensic scientist — a procedure not possible to the original Commission which had no forensic scientists as members of the Commission or staff. Indeed the Commission saw no need for advice and consultation by any forensic science specialist in its deliberations.

The procedure used in this book starts with the Commission's own data and then evaluates the information according to accepted standards of the forensic science profession.

New information, released under painful conditions by the National Archives, is from time to time referred to in the book. Its weight and relevance can be judged by the reader.

Secrecy

Much damage has been done to the credibility of the Warren Commission Report and to the credibility of the individual members of the Commission by the stubborn and irrational iron curtain of secrecy that has been pulled over the files of the

Commission. Even key witnesses who were to present crucial evidence under oath were denied access to material evidence that they themselves had generated. For example, the autopsy pathologists, in a proper routine fashion according to the best practices of the profession, made numerous color photographs of the late President's body; these exposed pictures were then spirited away (undeveloped) by Secret Service agents. They were not viewed by the pathologists in preparation for their testimony, nor were they admitted in evidence as integral exhibits in the complete testimony of the pathologists who actually had performed the autopsy. This situation was contrary to published federal directives.

Later attempts on the part of experts to study these photographs have been thwarted by unjustified and unjustifiable secrecy.

In producing this screen of secrecy, resort to lies has been commonplace. The Report gave the impression that the Commission did not have access to the photographs and wanted no such access. Later a forcing into the open of some minutes of an executive secret session of the Commission demonstrated that at least one photograph was available to the Commission and that it caused much confusion among the Commission members and staff.

Federal judges have been in collusion with federal executive officials in denying access to public documents connected with the case. The federal courts have cooperated in twisting legal definitions and interpretations to the end of circumventing the clear provisions of the Freedom of Information Law. The desperate attempts of these various officials to keep as many of the records of the Warren Commission as possible "under wraps" is clear indication that there is substantial material that must be suppressed in order to avoid embarrassment to officials, agencies, or citizens in high places.

The plea of national security as an argument in favor of continued secrecy is silly and dishonest. The number of documents in the entire federal collection that could possibly compromise national security is minute. The vast bulk of "classified" paper is so designated in order to hide official stupidity or wrongdoing, to give status to an otherwise pedestrian document or originator, for administrative convenience, or for raw political reasons having nothing to do with national security.

If opened, the files on the John F. Kennedy murder could in no way jeopardize national security, especially after the passage of over a decade since the files were accumulated. Official misbehavior might be revealed. Ineptitudes, incompetence, and other forms of "clay feet" attached to some public figures might see the light of day. The nation would be better for such exposure; she would be stronger. The people know it. It is probably true that most of the "secrecy guards" know it. They persist in their misbehavior for reasons obscure to most honest and rational citizens.

Is it any wonder then that the conclusions of the Warren Commission are looked on with skepticism by most Americans and as a sick joke by most thinking foreigners? The corrosive effects of this disbelief in federal reports and statements have been amplified by the reinforcing effect of the Watergate scandals and the questionable validity of a number of other reports that have come from federal sources by "blue ribbon" commissions.

Hopefully, some progress can be made in restoring the faith of Americans in their central government. The place to start is with the sad record of the investigation of the murder of President John F. Kennedy. The entire episode and its so-called investigation need reappraisal. In this book, only the medicolegal aspects of the case will be examined in order to show that there is ample reason, on that basis alone, to make a thorough "rerun" of what was one of the most tragic events in the twentieth century.

The Official View

It must be remembered that the official conclusion of the Warren Commission investigating the murder of John F. Kennedy was that the late President was shot from the rear by an individual named Lee Harvey Oswald who acted alone, with no accomplice and no advisors. Oswald was said to have been standing at a window on the sixth floor of a building known as the Texas School Book Depository. The investigating Commission concluded that there was no conspiracy of any kind involved in the President's murder.

The Commission also maintained that three shots and three shots only were fired. The Commission concluded that the first shot went into President Kennedy's back and out his throat. Then in some way that same bullet is claimed to have made two turns in midair and to have inflicted wounds on Governor Connally on the extreme right of his chest. The second bullet is said to have entered the President's brain, destroying it and a good portion of his skull and killing him instantly. The third shot has never been accounted for.

The various arguments and theories with respect to what actually happened are secondary to the most critical question, which involves where the bullets did, in fact, enter the President's body, how many bullets actually were fired, and where any of these bullets exited. The key question of the John F. Kennedy assassination is connected to the physical evidence. Physical evidence should show where the bullets came from, where they struck the President, and what organs and tissues were actually destroyed in the process. A bullet entrance hole in skin is usually not too difficult to identify. It is ordinarily round in outline and shows a number of unique characteristics. It is somewhat smaller than the diameter of the bullet because the skin tends to contract after the bullet passes through it. The exit hole is usually larger than the entrance hole because the bullet may be tumbling. However, the exiting bullet tends to clip and tear tissue and to push bits of tissue, bone, and other material in front of it as it passes out through the skin.

According to Gee (1968), entrance bullet wounds made at a range of over 2 feet appear "as a round hole with a band of abrasion around the margin of the hole, about 1/16 inch broad." If the bullet has been lubricated by a greaselike material, there will be, outside the abrasion, a rim of grease soiling on the skin. Copper-jacketed bullets do not show the rim of soiling. On the other hand, an exit wound made by a bullet is ordinarily in the form of an irregular split or tear. Margins are everted. There is no soiling of the neighboring tissue.

In clothing, the entrance hole of a bullet is regular. If the entrance of the missile is perpendicular to the surface, the fibers will be cut precisely. If the bullet hits at an acute angle, the cloth is frayed and then the hole is made. Little of value can be said about an exit hole in cloth other than that the torn fibers are pointed outwardly. As a rule of thumb, a split, flap-like, irregular tear is more characteristic of an exit through cloth than it is of a long-range entrance hole (Ceccaldi, 1962).

It is also important to understand that bullets frequently carry traces of foreign substances picked up in the passage through the body or inanimate structure. Microscopic and serological examinations may reveal fragments of liver, brain, muscle, fibrous tissue, and the blood type of the body from which the fragment came. Microchemical analyses can reveal plaster, cement, or metal traces picked up by a bullet.

According to Spitz and Fisher (1973), a diagnostic sign of a bullet entrance hole is "circumferential marginal abrasion," caused by scraping of the margins of the hole by the passing bullet. If the bullet strikes the skin perpendicularly, the scraping by the bullet is equal all around the margin. If the bullet strikes at an angle, the hole is round; the marginal abrasion is oval in outline.

Marginal abrasion of an exit wound is rare. It may occur when the bullet exits through skin which is held in place by tight-fitting clothing.

A dirt ring is seen around the marginal abrasion when the bullet is lubricated with greasy material.

Generally, exit wounds conform to no set pattern.

These facts summarized are well known to forensic scientists. They are not strange and unusual matters that could be easily overlooked by homicide investigators.

The Armed Forces Institute of Pathology has published basic, reliable information on the characterization of gunshot wounds and on the effective way to interpret gunshot wounds (Young and Stahl, 1966).

A serious error associated with gunshot wound investigation is "failure to perform a complete autopsy." The value of the clothing overlying a gunshot wound is shown to be at times crucial in deciding whether a hole is an entrance or an exit wound. This fact is a matter of common knowledge among competent homicide investigators.

Finck (1966) has emphasized "the abrasion ring is characteristic for a wound of entry."

Microscopic examination of skin edges around a bullet entry wound often shows elongated pycnotic nuclei. Foreign material and cellular debris may be dragged into the entry wound. If clothing overlaid the entry wound, fibers of the fabric may be identified in the entry wound. In many entry wounds, collagen and striated muscle fibers show an obvious fuchsinophilic necrosis (Finck, 1966).

Damage to collagen fibers in the entry wound stain red in Masson stain; they show marked birefringence. Elongated packed epidermal nuclei are common at the edge of the entry wound, a phenomenon named "streaming" (Adelson, 1961). Streaming identifies microscopically a wound of entry.

The microscopic examination of the bullet wounds in President Kennedy's remains did not include observations of these critical characteristics.

The Current Situation*

Despite massive efforts by the United States Information Service to "sell" the Warren Report on the Kennedy assassination to other nations, most foreigners doubted that the incident was carried out by one man unaided. These doubts have increased with time until the vast majority of American citizens by the mid-1970s express no confidence in the report of the Warren

---

*Meunier (1976) has published a short volume which brings together the questionable aspects of the entire investigation in the hope that a meaningful review of the matter *in toto* will be made. Meunier's book is marred at times by careless language. Nevertheless his book makes a strong case for a thorough reevaluation of the John F. Kennedy murder. Such a study will require the utmost care to insure free access to *all* material evidence in the case.

Commission.*

The study presented in this book will examine the medicolegal information which is part of the Report, the Hearings, and the Exhibits. The accepted, routine, mandatory details of a forensic autopsy will be discussed. The federal regulations covering such autopsy procedure will be reviewed. Then what actually transpired will be compared with what ought to have been done.

Finally, the author's conclusion will be presented after making a critique of the various medicolegal ramifications of the case.

The Select Committee on Assassinations

As of April 1977, the House of Representatives' Select Committee on Assassinations was still in a chaotic state. A chairman of the Committee has resigned, the chief counsel for the Committee had been forced to resign under pressure, and the prospects for useful and reliable information resulting from the Committee's endeavors were hazy.

In March 1977, the Committee had questioned Santos Trafficante, Jr., a reputed Mafia leader, about information he might have had concerning the murder of John F. Kennedy before the event occurred.

The Committee had been previously instructed that Trafficante would refuse to answer all such questions under his Fifth Amendment rights. Because of previous court decisions covering the use of the Fifth Amendment rights, Trafficante's lawyers were faced with a serious dilemma. If their client answered a single question, even one or two harmless questions, he could be found guilty of contempt of Congress if he did not answer

---

*An interesting preview of the Warren Commission Report is found in the *New York Times* page 1, 1 June 1964. A feature by Anthony Lewis has the headline, "Panel to Reject Theories of Plot in Kennedy Death." In an exclusive news story printed about three months before the Warren Commission finished taking testimony and four months before the Report saw the light of day, the *New York Times* printed the gist of it. Had the Commission made up its collective mind before all the data were collected? Numerous questions arise from this fact, especially since all the Commission operations were supposed to be closed until the Report was published.

all the questions. The strange rulings that came in part from the hysterical days of the Joseph McCarthy era, in a sense, deny the right of an individual to be selective concerning the Fifth Amendment during his testimony. Therefore, it is understandable how lawyers would recommend to a client that the safest course is to refuse to answer all the questions.

Despite the clear warning that Trafficante would stand upon his Fifth Amendment rights, the Committee, in a public hearing, went through a litany of fourteen questions on the subject. Trafficante refused to answer all questions. The session of the Committee was clearly not productive; one wonders why the energies of the Committee were wasted in following a course of action known, before the fact, to be ineffective. The echos from the Joseph McCarthy era are too loud to be amusing.

The Committee has also released three so-called "leads" that are claimed to justify further support of the investigation. Apparently the release of these items of information has been effective, at least in getting three years of additional life for this particular committee. One item is an obscure memo from the late J. Edgar Hoover. The memorandum speculatively has been claimed as evidence that the Central Intelligence Agency did, in fact, lie to the Warren Commission. A second item involves an unnamed nurse in the emergency room at Parkland Memorial Hospital in Dallas, Texas, where Governor Connally was treated for his serious gunshot injuries. It is claimed that she said there was too much lead removed from the Governor to agree that his wounds were caused by the magic, undeformed bullet found on an unattended stretcher in Parkland Hospital.

It seems that before passing out such frivolous stories, the Select Committee members would do well to read the twenty-six volumes of the Warren Commission Report. In that Report, the sworn statements of the three pathologists who performed the John F. Kennedy autopsy are printed. All three unanimously testified that the single, magic bullet could not have done the damage attributed to it by the Warren Commission. That Commission refused to accept the sworn testimony of its own expert pathologists.

What possible serious value can the statement of a nameless emergency room nurse have in the face of the sworn professional opinions of three certified pathologists, one of whom, Doctor Finck, is a fellow of the American Academy of Forensic Sciences?

The complexion of the House Select Committee is unpromising. Forensic Science competence on the Committee or its staff seems to be stubbornly lacking. It is bewildering to serious students of the John F. Kennedy murder why the Warren Commission saw fit to exclude any forensic science competence from its make-up. Apparently the Select Committee is also determined to exclude any forensic science competence from its membership.

On the basis of the performance, the attitudes, and the personnel of the House Select Committee on Assassinations as of April 1977, it is reasonable to hold that little of value will be realized from the Committee's activities.

Will we ever know the truth, the whole truth, and nothing but the truth in this matter? The author is pessimistic. On the other hand the ghost of a murdered President will not rest until the facts of his brutal, untimely death have been sorted out and evaluated as honestly as man can accomplish at this time and under the conditions which obtain with respect to the extant evidence.

CHAPTER 2

THE FORENSIC AUTOPSY

THE forensic autopsy (medicolegal autopsy) is distinctive in its goals and impact. One goal is to establish the cause of death. In addition, however, the autopsy must address itself to a clear identification of the body. The time of death must be looked into; evidence of foul play must be documented; the presence of poisonous agents in the body must be established or their absence demonstrated; the manner of death must be recorded (accidental, homicidal, suicidal, natural). The hospital type autopsies are merely for the purpose of confirming or modifying a previous clinical diagnosis.

The implications associated with the results of a forensic autopsy are numerous, complicated, and often unexpected until a challenge arises. Months or even years after the forensic autopsy is completed, insurance problems may surface, inheritance complications may demand the autopsy results, or prosecution of a felony may crystallize. In even the cases that appear innocent or those in which, on the surface, the cause and manner of death are obvious, it is imperative that a complete autopsy be performed; too often the routine cases ultimately turn out to be difficult.

A concise but thorough description of the scene of a homicide is mandatory for an adequate forensic autopsy. Sketches and photographs are of extreme importance in any such description. These data are properly part of the forensic autopsy report.

External Description of the Body

First the clothing is described and listed in a complete inventory. Sketches, measurements, and photographs all belong as part of the clothing description. Bullet holes in jackets or shirts must be described in words and illustrated by precise sketches and photographs. Color film is so cheap that its use in autopsies should be routine. For each hole in a piece of clothing, there must be a description of whether the fibers are bent inward or outward; a hand lens aids in such examination. Are there soot or powder marks around the holes? If so, what is the density and distribution of the foreign particles? How much blood is on the clothing? What is its distribution?

Needless to say, the autopsy report should clearly indicate whether the body was fully clothed, partially clothed, nude, or in a body bag. As the clothing is examined, the autopsy pathologist must work downward, layer by layer, removing each garment one by one, until the body is completely unclothed. The condition of each layer of clothing is precisely described before that layer is removed. Photographs and sketches that show precise sizes and relationships are critical and should be included to illustrate the autopsy report.

The body of President Kennedy was apparently received by the pathologists unclothed and wrapped in sheets. The precise sequence of events involved in disrobing the body is obscure. Who, when, how, and where are not obvious. What happened to the Ace® bandage that Arlen Specter seemed so concerned about in his interrogation of witnesses? What was the disposition of the late President's body brace? The chain of custody of various items of clothing is not a matter of record.

In any forensic autopsy performed according to ordinary standards of competence, the victim's body is delivered to the pathologist with the clothing on it. The pathologist then removes the clothing in an orderly fashion.

This routine practice was not carried out during the autopsy on the remains of late John F. Kennedy.

Sex, age, and race are recorded. Fingerprints should be taken and made a part of the autopsy record so that there will never in the future be a question about the identity of the victim. There is no record of the fingerprints of President Kennedy's corpse made at the autopsy.

The size of the body is recorded in terms of length, weight, general appearance with respect to nourishment, and other aspects that indicate how big the victim was, e.g. large bones, thick ankles. If any malformations are visible they are described in detail and photographed.

Is rigor mortis present? If so, how far advanced? Is livor mortis present? If so, what is the distribution and degree? The body temperature should be recorded if the body has been recently brought from the scene. In any case of importance a record of the rectal temperature should be routine.

Degree of clouding of the cornea is recorded, as is eye and hair color. Head hair pattern is described and, if noteworthy, a special sketch or photograph is made to show a unique feature that may be present. Conjunctivae of the eyes are described, whether pale, congested, or showing petechial or other kinds of hemorrhages. The location, size, and description of significant scars, tattoos, moles, or other external identifying marks must be clearly specified. Any evidence of external injuries must be included. Is the injury due to blunt force? Is it due to a knife or other sharp instrument? Are there bruises or abrasions? Are there small lacerations? Are they postmortem or premortem?

What is the condition of the external genitals? Is there anything noteworthy? For example, was the victim circumcized or not? Are varicocoele present?

In any important case an exact dental chart is appropriate. For all unknown and unidentified bodies, such a complete dental chart is mandatory.

All external evidence of disease must be included in the report.

A gunshot wound of the skin or other external portion of the body is described and the entire wound tract delineated in a single separate section of the autopsy report. No responsible pathologist fails to dissect carefully and completely the entire wound track in any missile wound case. Entrance and exit wounds are clearly indicated in words, sketches, photographs, and measurements. These data are an integral part of the autopsy report, which must be considered defective without them. Samples of tissue from the exit and entrance wounds are collected for microscopical study and for microchemical analyses. The path of the missile is described with reference to the planes of the body. The track is described in order as it moves through various anatomical parts. The injuries to the organs traversed by the missile are described clearly and measured in inches or millimeters. The thickness of each organ traversed is recorded. Photographs and sketches are obviously critical in such complete descriptions. Without these illustrations the autopsy report is defective.

The entrance and exit wounds are described in such detail as to obviate any future confusion. Marginal abrasions, powder marks, soot, and other material associated with the wounds must be clearly and fully described. Photographs of the abrasions are of extreme importance in helping to document the probable direction from which the missile entered the body.

A sample description of a bullet path is as follows. "The bullet track through the body goes from front to back, from right to left, and slightly upward."

Both exit and entrance wounds are located on the body by the length of a line from the top of the head and another line from the midline of the body (the neural crest of the vertebrae). Local landmarks on the body may be useful, e.g. a nipple, the navel. A bullet wound is never probed with any object until a definite conclusion has been made whether the wound is an entrance (inshoot) or an exit (outshoot). In describing a missile wound the term *perforated* is used to refer to a wound that has an entrance and an exit in an organ (it is a through-and-through wound). The term *penetrated* refers to one with an entrance wound only; there is no exit of the missile from the organ.

Internal Examinations

In the forensic autopsy, the internal examination must include a complete description of the head for injuries and any pathology that may exist in the brain structures. The neck is dissected carefully to explore the soft tissues as well as the cartilages in the neck. The spinal column in the neck region must also be evaluated.

The body cavities (chest and belly) should be described with respect to amount of fat, free fluid in the cavities, gross variations of any organs from normal range, any evidence of injuries, hemorrhages whether large or small, and any other observation that might be apparent.

The cardiovascular system (heart and blood vessels) must be evaluated in detail including a thorough dissection of the heart with the taking of samples for later microscopical study. Similarly, the respiratory tract study should include the weights of the lungs and their appearance, color and texture of the cut surfaces, location and description of any lesions no matter how small, the lymph nodes associated with the system, and the circulation of the lung area.

Intestinal tract examination includes the weights of the various organs, e.g. liver, pancreas, gall bladder. The appearance of the intact organ and of cut sections must be described. Any abnormalities or variations from normal range must be noted in adequate detail.

Kidney weight, appearance, and cut surface appearance are recorded. Male reproductive system is removed and described carefully; testes are cut across and cut surface described.

The endocrine glands, especially the thyroid, pituitary, and adrenals, are weighed, described, cut across, and samples are prepared for later microscopical examination.

Because elevated blood alcohol so frequently is found in both victims and perpetrators of violence, it should be a standard operating procedure to perform tests for alcohol content in the blood (or eye fluid if the blood cannot be obtained) of the victim being subjected to postmortem examination. Cases of outstanding importance (or if circumstances warrant) should include a drug screen for classes of drugs using liver, bile, brain, kidney, blood, or other samples as appropriate.

On a separate page the diagnosis or diagnoses were written. The major cause of death is listed as number 1. This page is then followed by the pathologist's opinion written in ordinary English; medical jargon should be avoided as much as possible. Virtually everyone who has any interest in the case will read this section of the autopsy report; it should be written with that fact in mind.

The opinion section should be concise, but all information that might be relevant to a court case must be included. Speculation has no place in this section. Keep to the point. The manner of death is stated clearly and without embellishment, i.e. homicide, accident, suicide, natural.

All supporting documents including preliminary sketches, notes, and memoranda are preserved in a file which can be used to back up the final written autopsy report if need be. Destruction of such back-up materials is professionally irresponsible.

Armed Forces Autopsy Procedures

In view of the fact that the autopsy of the murdered John F. Kennedy and all the associated examinations were controlled by the Department of Defense and its agents, it is informative to examine the standard procedures which are to be used in all postmortem examinations carried out under auspices of the Armed Forces. The autopsy of the late President Kennedy was carried out in a naval hospital by Army and Navy medical officers, physicians commissioned in these services as medical corps officers.

An official manual was and is available which "provides the prosector with ready and concise criteria on post mortem procedures and examinations" (Armed Forces Institute of Pathology, 1960). The point of this triservice manual is to provide a "directive toward uniformity in the selected techniques and objectives of an autopsy."

It would be expected that all commissioned officers who are pathologists in the medical services of the Armed Forces be thoroughly familiar with all details of this basic manual. Their military superiors would also have firsthand knowledge of the manual.

Two definitions as given in the official manual are pertinent to the Kennedy postmortem examination. "An autopsy is a scientific post mortem examination of a dead body, performed to reveal the presence of pathologic processes, their relation to clinical phenomena and history, and to determine the cause or causes of the changes encountered" (Armed Forces Institute of Pathology, 1960, p. 2).

In the manual, a medicolegal autopsy is recognized as having unique requirements which are spelled out in another definition, that of the medicolegal autopsy. "A specialized type of autopsy authorized or ordered by proper legal authorities in cases of accidental, suicidal, homicidal, unattended, or unexpected deaths in order to protect society and insure justice for the purpose of determining the cause of death."

One might question whether proper legal authority did in fact authorize the autopsy on President Kennedy. Regardless of that question, it is safe to assume that the pathologists who actually performed the autopsy thought that they were operating under proper legal authority and were empowered to carry out all warranted procedures without reference to next of kin or other interested persons.

Therefore, the instructions given in the manual are important with respect to the extent of the autopsy. "Whatever type of autopsy is performed, the examination should not be restricted to only those situations which are the seat of obvious alteration, but should include all organs of the body, for the normality of certain viscera is often as significant as the disease of others, and organs that appear normal macroscopically are frequently abnormal microscopically."

A thought-provoking directive is contained in this official manual. "Authority of officers and employees of the military services to conduct autopsies must derive from regulations or other directives of the military service concerned." It would be of interest to know what regulations or directives were operative at the time of John F. Kennedy's death to cover the autopsy on a civilian chief of state, killed in a civilian jurisdiction, in a nonmilitary situation. At least there is clear evidence that the autopsy performed had to meet the requirements peculiar to a medicolegal examination; of that there could have been no doubt on the part of the pathologists or of any other commissioned officers, no matter how high a rank, who may have been involved in any way in the postmortem examination.

In Appendix A are the complete directions for performing a general autopsy as outlined in the military manual. It is apparent that *every* organ must be examined in detail and that microscopic slides are prepared of all organs (after appropriate preparation and processing) for detailed study to reveal information not disclosed by gross examination.

SPECIAL PROCEDURES AND DIRECTIONS
FOR A MEDICOLEGAL AUTOPSY

In this following section is contained a verbatim reproduction of general precautions to be observed in the performance of a medicolegal autopsy in any of the Armed Forces establishments of the United States. The directions apply to *all* military pathologists performing such postmortem examinations. The quality of the final product depends in large part on how well the pathologists involved carry out the study in conformity with the official manual, which was prepared at the world-renowned Armed Forces Institute of Pathology.

Special Evidentiary Objectives of the Medicolegal Autopsy

GENERAL PRECAUTIONS TO BE OBSERVED IN
THE PERFORMANCE OF A MEDICOLEGAL AUTOPSY

Preliminary Investigation with Civil Authorities

a. Before he performs the autopsy the pathologist should confer with the police, the investigating authorities, or others having information about the case, in order that he can recognize all available evidence. It should be a standing rule that neither the clothing nor the surface of the body be disturbed until examined by the pathologist. In no circumstances should the body be embalmed before performance of a medicolegal autopsy.

b. In the event the pathologist cannot visit the scene he should request a written preliminary report on the circumstances surrounding death from the investigating authorities prior to performing the autopsy. Photographs of the scene where the body was found and the photographs made by the pathologist should be attached to the final autopsy report.

c. Restrict witnesses to the autopsy to those whose presence is required either by law or to assist the pathologist.

d. Disclose information regarding the autopsy findings only to those who have a legal right to it.

Evidence

a. Have Photographs Made of all Potentially Important Evidence that can be Recorded Photographically. Photographs should be made in all medicolegal autopsies since they provide a valuable objective record.

b. Prepare detailed descriptions, diagrams, and measurements of all wounds or recent disturbance of the clothing or to the surface of the body.

c. A medicolegal autopsy should never be a partial autopsy and should always include the brain, spinal cord, and organs of the neck. X-ray examination of the extremities and vertebral column is essential if there is a reasonable chance that these structures may have sustained injury. The neck organs should always be examined since sudden death by suffocation can result from the presence of foreign bodies, particularly food, or fractures of the thyroid or cricoid cartilages.

d. Label all specimens removed from the body for further examination. Do not permit any interruptions in the continuity of custody of the specimens.

e. Blood for group determination should be taken routinely in deaths by violence in which blood has been shed. Blood and/or cerebrospinal fluid should be taken routinely for alcohol determination in all deaths from violence or unexplained causes.

f. Confine the historical part of the autopsy record to one section, the objective or factual part to another, and the interpretative or diagnostic to still another. Do not confuse what you have been told with what you have seen or with your opinions or diagnosis. The objective or factual part of the report should be prepared in such detail and clarity that the reader can form his own opinion of its significance. If any of your opinions or diagnoses are based to any degree on information supplied to you by others, this fact should be indicated in the report.

g. The medicolegal protocol must be correct in all dates, weights, measurements, and in spelling. The inch-pound measurements are preferable to the centimeter-gram. A single error lays the entire protocol open to the criticism of carelessness and may discredit the autopsy examination.

Objectives

The medicolegal autopsy has the special purpose of securing information needed for the administration of justice, even though such information is irrelevant by ordinary medical standards.

Special Problems

Some of the special problems of a medicolegal autopsy are the following:

a. *Are the Remains of Animal or Human Origin?* The remains may be so fragmentary or so extensively altered by post-mortem change that it is not immediately apparent whether they are human or animal.

> (1) If putrefactive changes are not too advanced the distinction can be made by means of the precipitin test. Specific antisera are available not only for distinguishing between materials of animal and human origin, but also for identifying the kind of animal from which the material was derived.
>
> (2) If the material to be identified includes any part of the bony skeleton, consultation with an anatomist, anthropologist, or roentgenologist will almost invariably establish or exclude human origin. The distinction between animal and human osseous tissue may be made by microscopic examination of a small fragment of bone. There are methods by which it is often possible to decide between animal or human origin of so small a trace as a single hair.
>
> (3) No matter how mutilated, decomposed, or burned the remains may be, it is highly probable that a complete and careful examination of them will yield information of medicolegal importance.

b. *The Identity of the Corpse.*

> (1) The medical investigator is responsible for arrange-

ments for the taking of photographs and finger prints in all instances in which identity is in doubt. If by reason of mutilation or putrefaction personal identity cannot be established by ordinary means, the investigator must procure all information which might conceivably be useful for this purpose.

(2) Evidence of sex, stature, age, and various inherent or acquired individual peculiarities may be obtained from the skeleton alone in the event that the evidence needed is not available from the soft tissues. Thus, the contour of the pelvis or skull of an adult usually makes it possible to recognize whether the remains are those of a male or female.

(3) When identification of a body or parts of a body is unusually difficult, or when multiple detached parts of several bodies present a problem, technical specialists are available to give aid as indicated in AR 638-42; BUMEDINST 5360.19; NAVMC 1129; and AFR 143-3. "When technical specialists are required to help in identification (in addition to those available in an area), field commanders will request certain designated headquarters, through channels, to furnish assistance. For example, an Army commander will request this assistance from the Quartermaster General; a Naval commander from the Bureau of Medicine and Surgery; or the Commandant of the Marine Corps and an Air Force commander from Air Material Command."

(4) Stature can be estimated with reasonable accuracy if the length of any one of the long bones of the extremities is known. Many skeletal features, including condition of the teeth, presence or absence of ossification centers, ossification of the cartilaginous plates between the epiphyses and diaphyses, closure of the endocranial sutures and presence of certain porotic or proliferative changes in the bones may provide information as to the age of the deceased. X-ray examination of an unidentified body may be useful for reasons other than disclosure of age. A large proportion of the adult population has had roentgenological examination at one time or another. That the

remains are those of a given missing person may be proved by comparison of post-mortem X-rays with those taken during life. In addition, X-ray studies may disclose evidence of bullets or other foreign bodies that might otherwise be overlooked.

(5) Evidence pertaining to identity of decomposed or mutilated remains is not confined to the skeleton. Surgical scars, healed fractures, disease processes may help to confirm or exclude the corpse as that of any specified missing person. Information as to the foods eaten at the last meal may prove of value in establishing identity.

c. Time of Death. All available sources of information should be utilized in determining the time of death. Knowledge of the time of death of a victim of homicide may prove that a given suspect could or could not be guilty. Three sources of information ordinarily relied upon are:

(1) *Witnesses.* Statements from witnesses who claim to have been present at the time of death, to have last seen the decedent alive or to have first seen the dead body. Such information may or may not be reliable and should never be depended upon to the exclusion of other sources of information.

(2) *Rate processes.* An approximation of the time of death can usually be made on a basis of knowledge of the length of time required for the onset or completion of any one or a combination of post-mortem changes. It is known that the temperature of a corpse tends to come into equilibrium with the temperature of its environment. Although the rate of this change is affected by many factors, the duration of the post-mortem interval may often be approximated by estimating the rate at which the body probably cooled. The factors which should be taken into consideration in making such an estimate include the size and state of nutrition of the body, whether it is nude or clothed and whether the environment is cold or warm. Measurements of the superficial and internal temperature of the body and the environmental temperature should be recorded. Other post-mortem changes

which occur at more or less predictable rates include livor mortis, rigor mortis, and the stage of putrefaction. The autopsy protocol should include a detailed account of all such post-mortem changes.

(3) *Associated events.* The time of death may be established in relation to certain other events which took place at a known time. For instance, if the ground under the body was dry even though rain had been falling for six hours when the body was found, the inference is that death had occurred before the rain started to fall. If an evening meal known to have been eaten by the decedent was found undigested in his stomach at autopsy, the inference is that death probably occurred before midnight. The number and kinds of associated events that may be useful in determining the time of death is infinite and their recognition and utilization depend on the alertness and imagination of the pathologist.

   d. Was the Fatal Injury Received at the Place in Which the Body Was Found?

(1) In the case of an unwitnessed death by violence it is likely to be of utmost importance to establish that the fatal injuries were or were not received at the place where the body was found.

(2) It may be obvious from the nature of the injuries that they could not have been inflicted without coincidental disturbances of the immediate surroundings. Injuries of such a nature as to indicate that death was preceded by a violent physical struggle would justify the assumption that they had been received elsewhere if the place in which the body was found was undisturbed. It may be apparent that the decedent bled from his wounds and if no blood is found at the place where the body was discovered, it can be assumed that the injuries were sustained at some other place. The distribution of livor mortis and rigor mortis should be carefully ascertained to determine if it is consistent with the position or attitude of the body as found. When a person is found dead as the result of mechanical violence, the medical investigator should view

the body and its environment before either has been disturbed.

e. Can the Probable Circumstances in Which the Fatal Injuries Were Received be Reconstructed by Examination of the Body and the Place Where it was Found?

(1) The distribution and character of blood drops or smears may be helpful in distinguishing between accident and assault. It may be of great importance to establish the direction from which the fatal injury was received. Thus, a wound of one type may be consistent with accident, whereas a wound of another type may provide clear evidence of assault. A wound in one location may be compatible with the defendant's plea that he acted in self-defense, whereas a wound in another may render such an allegation untenable. A single injury may be compatible with accident, whereas multiple injuries may in some circumstances be clearly indicative of deliberate assault.

(2) The character of the place where the body was found may indicate that the injuries were accidental or probably the result of assault. Thus, multiple injuries of a person found dead at the bottom of a ravine or on a highway may be consistent with death by accident, whereas the same injuries on a body found on the soft earth of a field could not be the result of an accident at that place.

(3) The nature and location of injuries are often the means of distinguishing between suicide and homicide. This is particularly true in the case of firearm injuries. In the study of fatal injuries of this kind, wounds of entrance must be distinguished from wounds of exit and the characteristics of the region of the entrance wound described in detail, for these indicate the distance between muzzle and target when the fatal shot was fired. Fouling of the disrupted tissues immediately beneath the entrance wound by powder residues indicates that the muzzle was in contact with the target at the moment of fire. Superficial fouling of the target by powder residues indicates that the muzzle was relatively close to the target. The shorter

the distance between muzzle and target the greater will be the tendency for the combustion residues to be concentrated in the immediate vicinity of the entrance wound. Rarely will combustion products be deposited on the surface of the target if range of fire is greater than eighteen inches. In cases of fatal injury by close range rifle or shotgun fire in which the question of suicide may be raised, two measurements should be made: The distance between the entrance wound and the trigger when the muzzle is placed against the wound, and the distance between the entrance wound and the forefinger of the extended hand. Such measurements will usually reveal whether the wound could have been self-inflicted. However, in certain instances of suicide the individual has been known to have used his toe or some external object in order to pull the trigger.

f. Is There Evidence of a Special Predisposition of the Deceased to Accidental or Suicidal Injury or to Assault?

(1) A rich source of information relating to special susceptibility to injury is provided by chemical examination of the blood, spinal fluid, or brain of the decedent for alcohol. A concentration indicative of acute alcoholism may make plausible an otherwise inexplicable accident. Acute alcoholism may account for suicidal dementia or for behavior changes likely to provoke assault.

(2) The presence of any one of a number of diseases which would predispose to unexpected collapse or to impairment of the normal protective mechanisms might serve to explain an otherwise obscure accident.

g. Is there Objective Evidence Relating to Time Elapsed Between Injury and Death? It may be of utmost importance from a medicolegal standpoint to establish as accurately as possible the interval between injury and death. Injury is usually followed by an orderly sequence of reactive changes, and a recognition of these may make it possible to estimate the time that has elapsed. Thus, microscopic examination of the injured tissues may show that a given injury could not have been sustained more than a few minutes before death or that injury was sustained hours, days, or weeks before death. The establishment of the civil or criminal responsibility of some individual may depend to a large degree upon the amount of care that has been exercised in the acquisition of such information. The circumstances may be such that a given individual could or could not be responsible for the fatal injury, if it were known that it was received before or after some specified time.

h. If There are Multiple Injuries, in What Sequence Were They Received? It is important not only to determine the interval between injury and death, but also to reconstruct the sequence in which any given series of injuries was received. In cases of multiple injuries, it may be found that certain wounds were received after others, some may even have been inflicted after death. In such instances it may be apparent that suicide or a plea of acting in self-defense is untenable. In other instances it may be found that the injuries were separated by hours or even days. If such injuries have resulted from assault, there may be clear evidence of premeditation and extreme cruelty.

i. Is There Evidence That More than One Assailant Participated in the Attack, and if so, What Injuries Can Be Attributed to Each? It is frequently impossible to determine whether one or several assailants participated in a given assault. Such a determination can be made, however, in many instances of homicide by shooting. If examination discloses that the injuries were inflicted by several different weapons as indicated by the character of the wounds or differences in bullets, it may sometimes be assumed that several persons participated in the attack. It is important not only that this fact be recognized but also that a detailed description be made of the extent and nature of the injuries produced by each assailant.

j. Were the Injuries Immediately Incapacitating and if not, to What Extent and for How Long Was the Deceased Capable of Movement?

> (1) It is important to interpret certain facts to determine the extent to which the decedent may have contributed to their existence. In such circumstances it may be important to know what he might have done after certain injuries were sustained. If he could not have come unaided to the place where his body was found, it can be assumed that someone is in possession of special knowledge regarding the circumstances in

which the injury was received.

(2) The distribution of blood stains may indicate considerable movement on the part of a wounded person. If the decedent was injured in a manner incompatible with further locomotion, it may be apparent that his assailant was also wounded.

k. Did the Assailant Leave Anything in or on the Body of the Victim that Might Assist in His Identification?

(1) Whenever one person injures another by means of physical violence it is probable that the assailant will leave something in or on the body of the injured person that will aid in the apprehension of the criminal. The most satisfactory evidence in this respect is provided by the finding of a bullet in the body of the dead person. A bullet frequently bears markings characteristic of the firearm from which it was discharged. Even though the bullet is not available, it may have left metallic traces in the skin or tissues by which its composition can be determined. If the bullet was fired from close range (under 18 inches), chemical or metallic residues are likely to be present on the skin or clothing of the wounded person. A bullet found in a body at autopsy should not be handled with forceps because of the introduction of artefactitious markings. Examination of residues may disclose not only the range of fire but also the nature of the ammunition that was used. In the absence of the bullet, the ejected shell case may provide valuable evidence as to the identity of the weapon.

(2) Wounds should be examined before the body is moved, and if it is apparent from the entrance wound that the bullet was jacketed and probably from an automatic pistol, a search should be made for the empty shell case before the body is moved. A marginally soiled entrance wound may constitute presumptive evidence that the bullet was fired from a revolver, whereas a clean entrance wound sometimes indicates that the bullet was fired from an automatic pistol or rifle. Tissue for histopathological examination should be taken from the entrance wound.

(3) The shape or configuration of wounds may reveal the type of instrument used in their production. Thus, the pattern of an automobile tire or radiator grill may be imprinted on clothing or skin. Wounds produced by a given type of hammer, wrench, file, etc., may have highly individual characteristics. Such injuries should be photographed before and after the clothing has been removed and before and after the skin has been washed. Such photographs should either be of actual size or should be taken with a ruler laid close to the area being pictured.

(4) If there is evidence that the victim and his assailant engaged in a struggle, the latter may have been wounded and tests may disclose not only the blood group of the victim but also a different blood group of the assailant. Hairs of the assailant may be found in the hand of the dead person and abraded epidermis of the assailant may be found beneath the dead person's fingernails. In cases of fatal sexual attack in which rape has preceded or been coincident with murder, information useful in establishing the identity of the assailant may be obtained by testing the seminal fluid found on the person or clothing of the decedent. It may be possible to determine the blood group to which the assailant belongs even though the seminal stains are old and dry.

I. Is it Likely that Recognizable Traces of the Victim were Carried Away in or on the Person of the Assailant? It should be a routine procedure to determine the blood group of the victim of any kind of mechanical injury in which there is a possibility that blood from the decedent was transferred to the person of the assailant or to a weapon or instrument which the assailant may have taken from the scene of the attack. The finding on the clothing or on some article in the possession of a suspect of human blood to that of the deceased and unlike that of the suspect provides presumptive evidence either of guilt or incriminating knowledge.

The Brain

In any autopsy, but especially in a forensic autopsy, it is

imperative that the brain be removed from the skull and dissected with care. The official *Autopsy Manual* of the United States Armed Forces describes in detail the proper way to dissect and study the brain at autopsy. The material that follows is taken verbatim from that manual and is considered the usual and standard method of procedure for any autopsy.

Removal and Examination of the Brain

a. When bacteriologic or viral studies of brain tissue are indicated by clinical history or gross appearances, the brain should be removed prior to embalming.

b. After examination of the scalp, an intermastoidal incision extending over the vertex of the skull is made with the blade of the scalpel turned outward to prevent cutting the hair. If the subject is bald, the incision should be placed as far posteriorly as possible and may sometimes be hidden by making the incision backward from points about 2 inches above the ear to encircle the scalp posteriorly within the hairline. It is advisable to start the incision behind the right ear and end it behind the left, so that if disfigurement occurs, it will be on the left side of the head. Embalmers regard the right side of the face as the "show" side. Reflect the scalp anteriorly to a line 1.5 cm. above the supra-orbital ridge and posteriorly below the occiput. With a sharp instrument mark out the anterior saw cut from behind the ears over the frontal bone and, whenever possible, posterior to the hairline. The posterior cut should extend backward from the lower end of the anterior cut over the occipital bone to the midline at the level of the superior nuchal line, where it should meet with the posterior cut from the other side. The angle formed by the anterior and posterior skull incisions should be from 100° to 120° and should be so placed that neither limb, if extended, will intersect the external ear. This is of practical importance in protecting the ear from the saw. Use a scalpel to cut the temporal muscle and fascia along the plotted lines, and with a blunt instrument separate the tissues from the bone along the incision. Cut the entire thickness of the skull with a fine tooth saw or Stryker saw but do not allow the saw to slip into the brain. If there is a question of possible skull fracture, do not use hammer and chisel in removing the calvaria, as these implements may create fracture lines that will compli-cate medicolegal cases. Remove the calvaria, separating it from the underlying dura by blunt dissection between bone and dura. Open the superior longitudinal sinus. Cut the dura with scissors along the edges of the bone and reflect it toward the midline. Use scissors to cut the falx cerebri anteriorly in the great cerebral fissure and pull' the dura posteriorly, cut-ting the cerebral veins as necessary and the great cerebral vein of Galen in the pineal fossa. With the left hand lift the frontal lobes and olfactory nerves from the floor of the anterior fossa and use scissors to cut the optic nerves that can be reached. Place the left hand beneath the parietal lobes to support the weight of the brain and cut the tentorium cerebelli on each side beneath and close to its peripheral attachments. The posterior cranial fossa is exposed and the remaining cranial nerves and the vertebral arteries can be severed. Support the brain carefully with slight traction on the cerebral peduncles and transect the cervical cord as far inferioral as possible. Remove the brain by lifting it with the fingers of both hands to prevent damage to the soft organ.

c. After removal, fix the brain and spinal cord in 10 percent formalin. Before the brain is placed in fixative, the corpus callosum may be incised sagittally on each side of the midline to permit access of fluid to the ventricles. Suspend the brain in a gallon jar of fixative by a string passing under the basilar artery and attached to the edges of the container. The brain should be allowed to harden in fixative for at least one week, preferably two weeks, before sectioning. The fixing fluid should be changed during the first 24 hours and at the end of one week. If immediate diagnosis is necessary, the brain may be cut in the fresh state. This procedure is expedited if the freshly sectioned surface is pressed firmly against a piece of glass before the next cut is made, and the knife blade is flooded with 95 percent alcohol. If desired, the intact fixed brain may be forwarded to the Armed Forces Institute of Pa-thology.

d. When the brain has hardened in fixative it should be cut in coronal sections not more than 1 cm. in thickness. Place the brain on a dissection board with the ventral surface up-ward so that the landmarks of the base can be used in orienting the coronal cuts symmetrically. Remove the brain stem and cerebellum with a thin knife, cutting across the cerebral peduncles in a plane perpendicular to the axis of the brain stem and aqueduct. Begin the parallel coronal sections of the cerebral hemispheres at the frontal poles. The brain stem and cerebellum together are cut by parallel sections 0.5 cm. apart in a plane perpendicular to the axis of the brain stem.

Examination of the Base of the Skull

a. Fractures of the Base. For demonstration of fractures the dura should be stripped from the bone. This is best done by winding it onto a hemostat attached to the cut edge of the dura. Some pathologists prefer to use "gas pliers." In either case the dura should be stripped immediately after the brain is removed and before chisel and hammer are used, since they may cause fractures.

The autopsy report on John F. Kennedy stated that the skull was extensively fractured; it apparently came apart in the hands of the pathologists. There is no evidence in the Report that the skull fractures were studied as directed in the official *Autopsy Manual.* What might have been revealed by such a study is a matter of conjecture.

Some Implications

The Armed Forces *Autopsy Manual* provides a *directive.* That term clearly means that military establishments and personnel *will* carry out the indicated procedures because they are, officially and in writing, considered to be the minimal acceptable level of performance as determined by the average performance standards of the profession and any unique demands of the military service and must be performed as the procedures of choice.

The manual does not claim to provide "guidance," which is merely an outline or series of suggested things to do. It provides a directive — an exposition of what military pathologists are *directed* to do.

Additional tests and procedures may of course be added, if the pathologist in charge deems such to be necessary, but only after the minimal standards have been accomplished.

Extent of the Autopsy

There is no support in military regulations or directives for the so-called partial autopsy; standards of medical excellence do not look with approval on such incomplete evaluations. The directive under which military installations and personnel must perform autopsies is unequivocal concerning the extent of an adequate autopsy. Regardless of the kind of autopsy performed, even a routine hospital autopsy, the examination must not be limited to the obvious. The directive emphasizes that *all* organs must be examined because too often the obvious is misleading. Moreover, the need of microscopical examination of organs and tissues is stated clearly.

The official military directive for all personnel and installations involved in autopsies of any kind is that *all* organs *will* be examined and reported and that microscopical examinations *will* be performed as well as gross studies. Photographs and x-rays are considered essential and integral parts of the autopsy report, not merely appendices, addenda, or afterthoughts.

It is obvious, therefore, that to meet the minimal standards of acceptable performance for autopsies as demanded by Armed Forces directives the following organ systems in the male will be examined, grossly and microscopically, and the results will be reported in the autopsy write-up.

a. Nervous system (brain and spinal cord)
b. Cardiovascular system (heart and major vessels as well as vessels in the vicinity of any lesions)
c. Digestive system (esophagus, stomach, intestines, rectum, liver, gall bladder, pancreas)
d. Respiratory system (mouth, nasal passages, trachea, larynx, bronchi, lungs)
e. Endocrine system (thyroid, parathyroids, adrenals, gonads, pituitary)
f. Musculoskeletal system (x-rays to reveal skeletal condi-

tion; samples of muscle for microscopical study)
g. Skin
h. Spleen, lymph nodes, auditory apparatus, bone marrow
i. Genitourinary system (kidneys, bladder, testes, prostate, urethra, associated structures)

An autopsy that covers less than the above is by Armed Forces standards inadequate, incomplete, and not in compliance with written directives. From the broader point of view, it is not in accord with the minimal standards demanded by the forensic science profession.

Authority

The authority governing the conducting of autopsies by military pathologists derives unequivocally from written regulations and directives. These regulations and directives bear the seal and force of the service concerned; individuals, no matter what their rank, have no right to flout these directives nor to attempt to force others of lower rank to defy the letter, spirit, and intent of the directives and regulations. To do so is to commit a serious infraction of military regulations.

Persons outside of the Armed Forces have no authority to intrude in the execution of proper autopsy procedures by duly appointed military pathologists operating in military installations. Such intrusion should be adequate reason for arrest of the culprit by military authorities and the preferring of charges against the intruder.

Elementary common sense would force even a lukewarm military man or team to be completely familiar with all autopsy directives and regulations and to carry out an autopsy "by the book and by the numbers" when faced with the post-mortem investigation of a death of national, indeed international, concern. A performance that is any less than that demanded by clear-cut regulations demonstrates unbelievable stupidity or the involvement of forces beyond the control of the military pathologists concerned and operating counter to the best interests of medicolegal science and thus of the nation.

Observers

Taylor (1974) has emphasized what still is the widely accepted attitude among professional pathologists toward "observers" at autopsies, especially forensic autopsies. "As few persons as possible should be in attendance while the autopsy is in progress. Only morgue assistants and the persons who are directly associated with the investigation should be present. The possibility of unfounded rumors, erroneous interpretations, and misunderstandings will be decreased by the exclusion of all but essential persons." The commotion produced by a bevy of onlookers makes an orderly, informative autopsy difficult if not impossible.

Summary
(Extracted from official Armed Forces *Autopsy Manual*)

DESCRIPTIVE PROTOCOL

General Instructions

a. Describe the body as a whole and each organ, avoiding the use of diagnostic terms. Include weights and measurements where indicated, and describe the shape, color, consistency, and natural surfaces of each organ, also lesions and malposition.

b. To facilitate processing at the Armed Force Institute of Pathology, Standard Form 503 (Autopsy Protocol) will be used.

c. A *clinical abstract* obtained from the clinical records or furnished by the clinician, and *clinical diagnoses* should be next in order and completed in the format indicated below. When death occurs outside of a hospital, a statement concerning the circumstances surrounding death should be included in the autopsy protocol in lieu of the clinical abstract. These statements should be furnished by investigating officers as prescribed in applicable regulations of the service concerned. In cases of *death from trauma,* the cause should be stated, e.g. gunshot wound, automobile accident, poison (kind), and the circumstances surrounding the death, such as homicide, suicide, accident, etc.

CLINICAL ABSTRACT

DATE OF ADMISSION:
COMPLAINTS:

    1. _____

    2. _____

    3. _____

HABITS: Alcohol, tobacco, narcotics, etc.

FAMILY HISTORY: List all information bearing on deaths, illnesses and hereditary tendencies.

PREVIOUS PERSONAL HISTORY: List all service in Army, Navy, or Air Force and duty in tropics.

PRESENT ILLNESS: Onset of present illness with chronologic abstract of illness.

PAST ILLNESSES: Include all illnesses, operations, wounds, venereal infections, and tropical diseases.

PHYSICAL EXAMINATION: Weight, height, temperature, pulse, respiration, and blood pressure. List all positive observations by systems.

LABORATORY AND X-RAY FINDINGS: Include *gross photographs,* and other pertinent materials, such as electrocardiographic interpretations or photographic copies of electrocardiograms, and significant X-ray films, or copies of these.

COURSE IN HOSPITAL: To include major therapeutic measures.

DATE AND HOUR OF DEATH:

CLINICAL DIAGNOSIS

These should be listed numerically on Standard Form 503, (Autopsy Protocol) as indicated in the following example:

Standard Form 503
Revised August 1954
Promulgated
By Bureau of the Budget
Circular A—32 (Rev.)

ROUTINE

CLINICAL RECORD	AUTOPSY PROTOCOL		

Date and Hour Died 8:26 A.M. P.M. 29 March 1958	Date and Hour Autopsy Performed 8:15 A.M. P.M. 31 March 1958	CHECK ONE		
		Full Autopsy	Head Only	Trunk Only
PROSECUTOR H. S. TRIPLER, CAPT., MC, USA	ASSISTANT	X		

CLINICAL DIAGNOSIS *(Including operations)*

1. Myocarditis of Unknown Cause.
2. Hypochloremia and Hyponatremia with Hypovolemia.
3. Cardiac Insufficiency, Secondary to Dg. 1 and Dg. 2.

PATHOLOGICAL DIAGNOSES

CARDIOVASCULAR SYSTEM:
1. Myocardial Hypertrophy, Idiopathic.
2. Interstitial Fibrosis.
3. Myocarditis, Focal, Chronic, Slight.
4. Atherosclerosis, Aorta, Minimal.

RESPIRATORY SYSTEM:
1. Chronic Passive Congestion.
2. Pulmonary Edema.
3. Atelectasis, Partial, Left Lung.
4. Interstitial Fibrosis, Left Lung.

SPLEEN AND HEMATOPOIETIC SYSTEM: Chronic Passive Congestion.

LIVER: 1. Controlobular Anoxia Necrosis.
2. Chronic Passive Congestion.

GALLBLADDER AND BILE DUCTS: None.

PANCREAS: Chronic Passive Congestion

GASTROINTESTINAL SYSTEM: Acute Duodenal Ulceration, Due to Candida Albicians.

GENITOURINARY SYSTEM: None.

ENDOCRINE GLANDULAR SYSTEM: None.   CENTRAL NERVOUS SYSTEM: None.

BONE AND JOINTS: None.   MISCELLANEOUS: Ascites.

APPROVED SIGNATURE
BURTON C. WALKER, Lt., MC, USA

MILITARY ORGANIZATION *(When required)*	Age 43	Sex M	Race Cau	Identification No. 366-08-00	Autopsy No. A-25-56
PATIENT'S IDENTIFICATION *(For typed or written entries give: Name-last, first, middle; grade; date; hospital or medical facility)*				Register No. 14807	Ward No. 10

COOKE, WYLLE M. Lt.
Washington Army Hospital, Mount Vernon, Virginia

AUTOPSY PROTOCOL
Standard Form 503

Gross Examination of Organs

a. Initial Procedure. Examine every organ in the body;
collect representative sections of each for histologic studies
and include skin, muscle, peripheral nerve, bone and marrow.

GENERAL: Approximate height and weight, age, color, sex,
condition as to development and nutrition, degree of rigidity, character and distribution of lividity and degree of
post-mortem decomposition. Detailed description of exte-
rior, beginning with hair and going to feet, including
marks of identification, superficial vessels, lymph nodes,
and external genitalia.

PRIMARY INCISION: Subcutaneous fat, muscles, peritoneum, omentum, subperitoneal fat, position and relations
of abdominal viscera, adhesions, fluid, intra-abdominal
and mesenteric lymph nodes; height of diaphragm; pleural
fluid; pericardium; thymus.

ORGANS OF NECK: Thyroid; parathyroids; larynx; pharynx.

LUNGS: Weight, relative size, consistency, pleura; cut surface
of each lobe; bronchi; hilum; lymph nodes.

HEART: Weight, relative size; epicardium; musculature;
valve leaflets; endocardium; coronary arteries; circumferential measurements of value orifices and thickness of ventricular walls.

AORTA AND VESSELS:

SPLEEN: Weight, size, consistency; capsule, cut surface;
color, dry or moist, markings; character of pulp.

LIVER: Weight, surface, consistency, color, and markings of
surface and parenchyma.

GALLBLADDER AND DUCTS: Contents; mucosa.

PANCREAS: Weight, consistency, cut surface.

ADRENALS: Size, cut surface.

GASTROINTESTINAL TRACT: Esophagus, stomach and
its contents; intestines; appendix.

GENITOURINARY TRACT: Kidney: Weight, size and consistency; capsule, subcapsular surface, cut surface; cortical
markings, width of cortex, pelvis, pelvic fat, ureter; large
vessels. Urinary bladder: amount and character of contents;
mucosa; wall.

SEMINAL VESICLES:

PROSTATE: or UTERUS, OVARIES AND ADNEXA:
TESTICLES:
HEAD: Scalp; calvaria; dura, blood sinuses of dura; lepto-
meninges, fluid or exudate; base of skull.
BRAIN: Weight, convolutions and sulci; cerebral blood ves-
sels; consistency; ventricles.
CORD: Dura; exudate; leptomeninges; appearance of cross
sections at representative levels.
TEMPORAL BONE:
EAR:
SINUSES OF SKULL:
EYES:
BONE MARROW: Ribs, sternum, vertebrae, shaft of femur
(when there is a hematologic problem).
MUSCLES:
BONES AND JOINTS:
BACTERIOLOGIC EXAMINATIONS:
CHEMICAL EXAMINATIONS:

b. Cause of Death. After completion of the gross autopsy
the pathologist should supply the attending physician with
the important pathologic diagnoses to aid him in establishing the cause of death. In some cases no anatomical cause
of death can be found at autopsy. In some cases subsequent
microscopic, chemical and bacteriological examination will
change the pathologic diagnosis. Such changes must be reported to the clinician or to the local bureau of vital statistics.
In the case of a medicolegal autopsy, the pathologist is responsible for determining the cause of death and uncovering
evidence which may be of legal importance.

Microscopic Description of Organs

HEART: Epicardium, epicardial fat, endocardium, myocardium, interstitial tissue, values, vessels.
LUNGS: Pleura, alveolar spaces, alveolar walls, interstitial
tissue, bronchi, vessels.
LIVER: Capsule, architecture, central areas, portal areas, interstitial tissue, fat hemorrhage, necrosis, pigment. *Gallbladder:* mucosa, wall.
PANCREAS: Acinar parenchyma, islets, ducts, vessels.

SPLEEN: Capsule, malpighian bodies, red pulp, trabecule, vessels.

ADRENALS: Cortex, medulla, tumors, vessels.

KIDNEYS: Glomeruli, tubules, interstitial tissue, vessels, pelvic mucosa.

PELVIC ORGANS:

   Bladder: Mucosa, submucosa, muscularis.

   Prostate: Glands, stroma, hyperplasia, inflammation.

   Seminal Vesicles: Mucosa, infection, concretions.

   Testes: Tubules, basement membrane, atrophy, spermatogenesis.

   Uterus: Endometrium, myometrium, tumors.

   Vagina: Mucosa and submucosa.

   Ovaries: Stroma, cysts, corpora albicantia and lutea, vessels.

LYMPHATIC SYSTEM: Capsule, architecture, follicles, stroma, pigment, reticulo-histiocystic components.

THYROID: Acini, stroma, degenerative changes.

BONE MARROW: Proportion of fat to hematopoetic elements. Normoblasts, myeloid elements, megakaryocytes. Hyperplasia or hypoplasia.

SKELETAL SYSTEM: Condition of trabecular bone, osteoblastic and osteoclastic activity.

BRAIN: Meninges, parenchyma, vessels, perivascular infiltrations, ependyma.

Final Summary of the Case (Epicrisis)

No autopsy protocol is complete without a final summary in which the prosector evaluates his findings and correlates them with the clinical history. Such an epicrisis should consist of:

   a. An abstract of about 100 words of the pertinent clinical history and of the clinical diagnostic problem. It should not duplicate the detailed clinical abstract which is furnished by the attending physician.

   b. A concise statement of the principal gross and microscopic observations at autopsy. This should not be a copy, but an abstract, of the diagnosis sheet.

   c. A discussion of the pathogenesis of the illness and the evolution of the structural changes which eventually led to death, based on the autopsy findings and the clinical history.

d. Where applicable, a discussion of the effects of therapy.

e. The prosector should state what he learned from the case or what the case should teach.

The Question

A decision on the quality and ultimate value of the autopsy performed on the remains of John F. Kennedy depends in great part on how well the actual examination conformed to the minimal standards set down for such procedures in the official Armed Forces autopsy directives. The following chapters concern themselves with such an evaluation.

CHAPTER 3

THE EVENTS OF THE MURDER

THE Report of the Warren Commission describes the murder of late President John F. Kennedy as follows (verbatim from the Report, pp. 1-4).

The assassination of John Fitzgerald Kennedy on November 22, 1963, was a cruel and shocking act of violence directed against a man, a family, a nation, and against all mankind. A young and vigorous leader whose years of public and private life stretched before him was the victim of the fourth Presidential assassination in the history of a country dedicated to the concepts of reasoned argument and peaceful political change. This Commission was created on November 29, 1963, in recognition of the right of people everywhere to full and truthful knowledge concerning these events. This report endeavors to fulfill that right and to appraise this tragedy by the light of reason and the standard of fairness. It has been prepared with a deep awareness of the Commission's responsibility to present to the American people an objective report of the facts relating to the assassination.

Narrative of Events

At 11:40 a.m., c.s.t., on Friday, November 22, 1963, President John F. Kennedy, Mrs. Kennedy, and their party arrived at Love Field, Dallas, Texas. Behind them was the first day of a Texas trip planned 5 months before by the President, Vice President Lyndon B. Johnson, and John B. Connally, Jr., Governor of Texas. After leaving the White House on Thursday morning, the President had flown initially to San Antonio where Vice President Lyndon B. Johnson joined the party and the President dedicated new research facilities at the U. S. Air Force School of Aerospace Medicine. Following a testimonial dinner in Houston for U.S. Representative Albert Thomas, the President flew to Fort Worth where he spent the night and spoke at a large breakfast gathering on Friday.

50

Planned for later that day were a motorcade through downtown Dallas, a luncheon speech at the Trade Mart, and a flight to Austin where the President would attend a reception and speak at a Democratic fund-raising dinner. From Austin he would proceed to the Texas ranch of the Vice President. Evident on this trip were the varied roles which an American President performs — Head of State, Chief Executive, party leader, and, in this instance, prospective candidate for reelection.

The Dallas motorcade, it was hoped, would evoke a demonstration of the President's personal popularity in a city which he had lost in the 1960 election. Once it had been decided that the trip to Texas would span 2 days, those responsible for planning, primarily Governor Connally and Kenneth O'Donnell, a special assistant to the President, agreed that a motorcade through Dallas would be desirable. The Secret Service was told on November 8 that 45 minutes had been allotted to a motorcade procession from Love Field to the site of a luncheon planned by Dallas business and civic leaders in honor of the President. After considering the facilities and security problems of several buildings, the Trade Mart was chosen as the luncheon site. Given this selection, and in accordance with the customary practice of affording the greatest number of people an opportunity to see the President, the motorcade route selected was a natural one. The route was approved by the local host committee and White House representatives on November 18 and publicized in the local papers starting November 19. This advance publicity made it clear that the motorcade would leave Main Street and pass the intersection of Elm and Houston Streets as it proceeded to the Trade Mart by way of the Stemmons Freeway.

By midmorning of November 22, clearing skies in Dallas dispelled the threat of rain and the President greeted the crowds from his open limousine with the "bubbletop," which was at that time a plastic shield furnishing protection only against inclement weather. To the left of the President in the rear seat was Mrs. Kennedy. In the jump seats were Governor Connally, who was in front of the President, and Mrs. Connally at the Governor's left. Agent William R. Greer of the Secret Service was driving, and Agent Roy H. Kellerman was sitting to his right (Fig. 3-1).

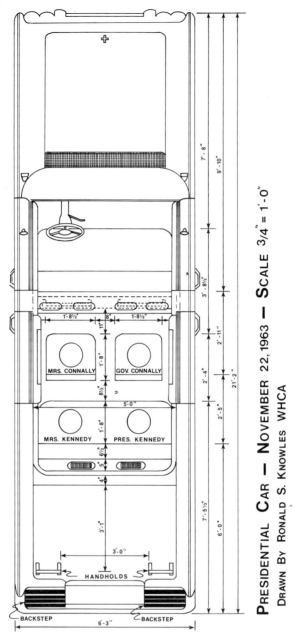

Figure 3-1. This is a diagram of the presidential limousine. It is a scale drawing and was published as Commission Exhibit Number 872 in volume 17 of the Hearings, page 867. The position of the President was directly behind that of Governor Connally. The relative positions of the two men make it improbable that a single bullet could have followed the path necessary to produce the wounds that the Warren Commission concluded had occurred.

Directly behind the Presidential limousine was an open "followup" car with eight Secret Service agents, two in the front seat, two in the rear, and two on each running board. These agents, in accordance with normal Secret Service procedures, were instructed to scan the crowds, the roofs, and windows of buildings, overpasses, and crossings for signs of trouble. Behind the "followup" car was the Vice-Presidential car carrying the Vice President and Mrs. Johnson and Senator Ralph W. Yarborough. Next were a Vice-Presidential "followup" car and several cars and buses for additional dignitaries, press representatives, and others.

The motorcade left Love Field shortly after 11:50 a.m., and proceeded through residential neighborhoods, stopping twice at the President's request to greet well-wishers among the friendly crowds. Each time the President's car halted, Secret Service agents from the "followup" car moved forward to assume a protective stance near the President and Mrs. Kennedy. As the motorcade reached Main Street, a principal east-west artery in downtown Dallas, the welcome became tumultuous. At the extreme end of Main Street the motorcade turned right on Houston Street and proceeded north for one block in order to make a left turn on Elm Street, the most direct and convenient approach to the Stemmons Freeway and the Trade Mart. As the President's car approached the intersection of Houston and Elm Streets, there loomed directly ahead on the intersection's northwest corner a seven-story, orange brick warehouse and office building, the Texas School Book Depository. Riding in the Vice President's car, Agent Rufus W. Youngblood of the Secret Service noticed that the clock atop the building indicated 12:30 p.m., the scheduled arrival time at the Trade Mart.

The President's car which had been going north made a sharp turn toward the southwest onto Elm Street. At a speed of about 11 miles per hour, it started down the gradual descent toward a railroad overpass under which the motorcade would proceed before reaching the Stemmons Freeway. The front of the Texas School Book Depository was now on the President's right, and he waved to the crowd assembled there as he passed the building. Dealey Plaza — an open, landscaped area marking the western end of downtown Dallas — stretched out to the President's left. A Secret Service agent riding in the motorcade radioed the Trade Mart that the President would arrive in 5 minutes.

Seconds later shots resounded in rapid succession. The President's hands moved to his neck. He appeared to stiffen momentarily and lurch slightly forward in his seat. A bullet had entered the base of the back of his neck slightly to the right of the spine. It traveled downward and exited from the front of the neck, causing a nick in the left lower portion of the knot in the President's necktie. Before the shooting started, Governor Connally had been facing toward the crowd on the right. He started to turn toward the left and suddenly felt a blow on his back. The Governor had been hit by a bullet which entered at the extreme right side of his back at a point below his right armpit. The bullet traveled through his chest in a downward and forward direction, exited below his right nipple, passed through his right wrist which had been in his lap, and then caused a wound to his left thigh. The force of the bullet's impact appeared to spin the Governor to his right, and Mrs. Connally pulled him down into her lap. Another bullet then struck President Kennedy in the rear portion of his head, causing a massive and fatal wound. The President fell to the left into Mrs. Kennedy's lap.

Secret Service Agent Clinton J. Hill, riding on the left running board of the "followup" car, heard a noise which sounded like a firecracker and saw the President suddenly lean forward and to the left. Hill jumped off the car and raced toward the President's limousine. In the front seat of the Vice-Presidental car, Agent Youngblood heard an explosion and noticed unusual movements in the crowd. He vaulted into the rear seat and sat on the Vice President in order to protect him. At the same time Agent Kellerman in the front seat of the Presidential limousine turned to observe the President. Seeing that the President was struck, Kellerman instructed the driver, "Let's get out of here; we are hit." He radioed ahead to the lead car, "Get us to the hospital immediately." Agent Greer immediately accelerated the Presidential car. As it gained speed, Agent Hill managed to pull himself onto the back of the car where Mrs. Kennedy had climbed. Hill pushed her back into the rear seat and shielded the stricken President and Mrs. Kennedy as the President's car proceeded at high speed to Parkland Memorial Hospital, 4 miles away.

At Parkland, the President was immediately treated by a team of physicians who had been alerted for the President's arrival by the Dallas Police Department as the result of a radio message from the motorcade after the shooting. The doctors noted irregular breathing movements and a possible heartbeat, although they could not detect a pulsebeat. They observed the extensive wound in the President's head and a small wound approximately one-fourth inch in diameter in the lower third of his neck. In an effort to facilitate breathing, the physicians performed a tracheotomy by enlarging the throat wound and inserting a tube. Totally absorbed in the immediate task of trying to preserve the President's life, the attending doctors never turned the President over for an examination of his back. At 1 p.m., after all heart activity ceased and the Last Rites were administered by a priest, President Kennedy was pronounced dead. Governor Connally underwent surgery and ultimately recovered from his serious wounds.

Upon learning of the President's death, Vice President Johnson left Parkland Hospital under close guard and proceeded to the Presidential plane at Love Field. Mrs. Kennedy, accompanying her husband's body, boarded the plane shortly thereafter. At 2:38 p.m., in the central compartment of the plane, Lyndon B. Johnson was sworn in as the 36th President of the United States by Federal District Court Judge Sarah T. Hughes. The plane left immediately for Washington, D.C., arriving at Andrews AFB, Md., at 5:58 p.m., e.s.t. The President's body was taken to the National Naval Medical Center, Bethesda, Md., where it was given a complete pathological examination.* The autopsy disclosed the large head wound observed at Parkland and the wound in the front of the neck which had been enlarged by the Parkland doctors when they performed the tracheotomy. Both of these wounds were described in the autopsy report as being "presumably of exit." In addition the autopsy revealed a small wound of entry in the rear of the President's skull and another wound of entry near the base of the back of the neck. The autopsy report

---

*The autopsy examination was not complete by any standards. The track of the nonlethal wound in the President's remains was not dissected and described. The brain was not dissected as it should have been, according to ordinary standards. The microscopic examination of the various tissues was superficial. (C.G.W.)

stated the cause of death as "Gunshot wound, head," and the bullets which struck the President were described as having been fired "from a point behind and somewhat above the level of the deceased."

On-the-scene News Stories.

Among the first reports of the wounds inflicted on President Kennedy and on Governor Connally was that of Merriman Smith, UPI White House reporter (United Press International, 1964).

He was in the press car that followed the presidential limousine to Parkland Hospital after the shooting. Immediately upon arrival at the hospital driveway, "Smith jumped from the press car and ran to the limousine."

"The President was face down on the back seat. Mrs. Kennedy made a cradle of her arms around the President's head and bent over him as if she were whispering to him."

Smith also observed the general conditions of Governor Connally at the time. He was on the car floor, on his back, his head and shoulders supported by his wife's arms. Smith wrote, "Blood oozed from the front of the Governor's shirt."

Smith further reported, "I could not see the President's wound. But I could see blood spattered around the interior of the rear seat and a dark stain spreading down the right side of the President's dark grey suit."

Smith remembered hearing three shots fired; the first sounded different than the other two, more like a large firecracker. Clint Hill, the Secret Service agent guarding Mrs. Kennedy, told Smith, while the late President still lay in the limousine, that Kennedy was dead.

The peculiar difference in the sound of the first shot has been referred to by a number of witnesses. A possible explanation is that defective ammunition (below usual power) was involved. Another explanation is that the first shot came from a significantly great distance and a different direction than did the others. Finally, a variation in the shot sound could well result from a different firearm and cartridge.

The United Press historical account describes the shooting as follows.

"At the crack of the shot, the President jerked sharply and clutched his neck. Governor Connally, sitting directly ahead of him, turned back toward the sound and was immediately tumbled into his wife's arms by a second shot. As Kennedy slumped forward, a third shot was fired."

The murder sequence took less than six seconds.

It is important to realize that the UPI story was based on immediate, eyewitness accounts. It was filed and printed before various interested persons could rethink what they wanted to see and before witnesses could forget, be bullied into modifying their statements, or be subconsciously influenced by what they later read and saw. As early eyewitness reports, these stories by the leading newsmen of the United States must be given great weight in any reevaluation of the incident. These stories, in relation to later data from analysis of motion picture films taken of the event and in the light of ballistics considerations, throw grave questions on the conclusions of the Warren Commission.

It is unfortunate that no tape recordings were available of radio or television programs covering the actual parade. The sound tracks would have recorded the exact number of shots and would have been available for analysis to reveal different qualities of each shot by spectrograph.

Early news reports contended that a nonfatal shot struck the President in the right shoulder below the collar by several inches; it was reported that the bullet had lodged in the body (*Washington Post*, 18 December 1963; *New York Times*, 26 January 1964). The *Washington Post* claimed (29 May 1966) that the FBI had confirmed before publication that the first bullet to hit President Kennedy was found deep in his shoulder.

New York Times

The first account of the late John F. Kennedy's shooting to appear in the prestigious *New York Times* was written by Tom Wicker on 23 November 1963. It disclosed that, as the presidential limousine was very near the triple underpass, a shot rang out; a first shot was said to have hit Kennedy. The news report went on to say that in response to the sound, Governor Connally turned in his seat and was immediately struck in the chest by another bullet. A crucial statement followed. "Mr. Kennedy was hit by a bullet in the throat just below the Adam's apple, they said (reference is to the emergency room doctors attending the stricken President) this wound had the appearance of a bullet's entry." Accounts like this one made soon after the event must not be discarded capriciously. Elapsed time is one of the most potent factors in rendering eyewitness testimony of questionable validity.

Early reports such as this one by Tom Wicker are more in keeping with the overall medicolegal data than are the actual conclusions of the Warren Commission.

Facts on File

Facts on File from the World News Digest (1963) stated that the late President Kennedy was hit in the head and in the neck by two bullets from a rifle fired by an ex-Marine, Lee Harvey Oswald. Three shots were said to have been fired; two hit President Kennedy. A third shot struck Governor Connally, who was wounded severely. The nonfatal bullet entered Connally's back, "smashed three ribs," punctured a lung, broke the Governor's wrist, and entered his left thigh.

Kennedy is reported to have become unconscious immediately upon being hit in the head. He died of a gunshot wound to the brain.

The body was flown back to Washington, D.C., and arrived at Andrews Air Force Base at approximately 6:00 PM EST.

Conclusions

The official conclusions concerning the details of the killing of Kennedy and the wounding of Connally are given verbatim below as the Warren Commission published (Report, pp. 18-19).

This Commission was created to ascertain the facts relating to the preceding summary of events and to consider the important questions which they raised. The Commission has addressed itself to this task and has reached certain conclusions based on all the available evidence. No limitations have been placed on the Commission's inquiry; it has conducted its own investigation, and all Government agencies have fully discharged their responsibility to cooperate with the Commission in its investigation. These conclusions represent the reasoned judgment of all members of the Commission and are presented after an investigation which has satisfied the Commission that it has ascertained the truth concerning the assassination of President Kennedy to the extent that a prolonged and thorough search makes this possible.

1. The shots which killed President Kennedy and wounded Governor Connally were fired from the sixth floor window at the southeast corner of the Texas School Book Depository. This determination is based upon the following:

(a) Witnesses at the scene of the assassination saw a rifle being fired from the sixth floor window of the Depository Building, and some witnesses saw a rifle in the window immediately after the shots were fired.

(b) The nearly whole bullet* found on Governor Connally's stretcher at Parkland Memorial Hospital and the two bullet fragments found in the front seat of the Presidential limousine were fired from the 6.5-millimeter Mannlicher-Carcano rifle found on the sixth floor of the Depository Building to the exclusion of all other weapons.

(c) The three used cartridge cases found near the window on the sixth floor at the southeast corner of the building were fired from the same rifle which fired the above-described bullet and fragments, to the exclusion of all other weapons.

(d) The windshield of the Presidential limousine was struck by a bullet fragment on the inside surface of the

---

*This expression is peculiar in its wording, which seems designed to mislead the reader. The bullet in question was virtually "pristine" and undeformed except for engraving of rifling marks and a slight lateral flattening of the base. The stretcher was never clearly shown to have been Connally's. (C.G.W.)

glass, but was not penetrated.

(e) The nature of the bullet wounds suffered by President Kennedy and Governor Connally and the location of the car at the time of the shots establish that the bullets were fired from above and behind the Presidential limousine, striking the President and the Governor as follows:

(1) President Kennedy was first struck by a bullet which entered at the back of his neck and exited through the lower front portion of his neck, causing a wound which would not necessarily have been lethal. The President was struck a second time by a bullet which entered the right-rear portion of his head, causing a massive and fatal wound.

(2) Governor Connally was struck by a bullet which entered on the right side of his back and traveled downward through the right side of his chest, exiting below his right nipple. This bullet then passed through his right wrist and entered his left thigh where it caused a superficial wound.

(f) There is no credible evidence that the shots were fired from the Triple Underpass, ahead of the motorcade, or from any other location.

2. The weight of the evidence indicates that there were three shots fired.

3. Although it is not necessary to any essential findings of the Commission to determine just which shot hit Governor Connally, there is very persuasive evidence from the experts to indicate that the same bullet which pierced the President's throat also caused Governor Connally's wounds.† However, Governor Connally's testimony and certain other factors have given rise to some difference of opinion as to this probability but there is no question in the mind of any member of the Commission that all the shots which caused the President's and Governor Connally's wounds were fired from the sixth floor window of the Texas School Book Depository.

4. The shots which killed President Kennedy and wounded Governor Connally were fired by Lee Harvey Oswald. This

---

†This statement is not accurate. If Connally was hit by a separate bullet, the lone assassin theory is not tenable; at least two shooters would be required. (C.G.W.)

conclusion is based upon the following:

(a) The Mannlicher-Carcano 6.5-millimeter Italian rifle from which the shots were fired was owned by and in the possession of Oswald.

(b) Oswald carried this rifle into the Depository Building on the morning of November 22, 1963.

(c) Oswald, at the time of the assassination, was present at the window from which the shots were fired.

(d) Shortly after the assassination, the Mannlicher-Carcano rifle belonging to Oswald was found partially hidden between some cartons on the sixth floor and the improvised paper bag in which Oswald brought the rifle to the Depository was found close by the window from which the shots were fired.

(e) Based on testimony of the experts and their analysis of films of the assassination, the Commission has concluded that a rifleman of Lee Harvey Oswald's capabilities could have fired the shots from the rifle used in the assassination within the elapsed time of the shooting. The Commission has concluded further that Oswald possessed the capability with a rifle which enabled him to commit the assassination.

Oswald's Marksmanship

The Commission stubbornly refused to recognize that Oswald, according to Marine Corps records, was an indifferent rifle shot. Once he barely qualified at the lowest level of competence recognized by the military. He held that low level only briefly. The clear fact, understandable to anyone who is familiar with riflery, is that Oswald's record proves him to have been a poor shot with the rifle; so poor indeed that he could not have performed the skillful shooting attributed to him (Report, p. 191) (Hearings, vol. 8, p. 304) (Hearings, vol. 11, p. 330).

It is not clear why the Commission felt compelled to force its conclusions into the lone assassin theory supported by the untenable postulate of one bullet's having wounded, nonfatally, both Kennedy and Connally.

The facts of Oswald's proficiency with a rifle argue against these conclusions.

The Commission Conclusions

The language of the conclusions is carefully chosen, a fact which seems to have escaped the eyes of many defenders of the Report as an adequate document. There is a clear air of uncertainty in the conclusions and a use of modifiers that arouses the concern of the analytical reader.

The Commission as a whole was dubious about the theory that one bullet inflicted the nonfatal wounds on Kennedy and Connally. Paragraph 3, page 19, of the Report presents the single bullet theory but claims that it "is not necessary to any essential findings of the Commission," a qualification that is hardly supported by all the evidence.

It is asserted vigorously, however, that the Commission unanimously and without question agreed that all the shots which struck Kennedy and Connally came from the sixth floor window of the Texas School Book Depository.

Further details of the actual shooting in the Commission's own words are given below (Report, pp. 48-52).

The Assassination

At 12:30 p.m., c.s.t., as the President's open limousine proceeded at approximately 11 miles per hour along Elm Street toward the Triple Underpass, shots fired from a rifle mortally wounded President Kennedy and seriously injured Governor Connally. One bullet passed through the President's neck; a subsequent bullet, which was lethal, shattered the right side of his skull. Governor Connally sustained bullet wounds in his back, the right side of his chest, right wrist, and left thigh.

The Time

The exact time of the assassination was fixed by the testimony of four witnesses. Special Agent Rufus W. Youngblood observed that the large electric sign clock atop the Texas School Book Depository Building showed the numerals "12:30" as the Vice-Presidential automobile proceeded north on Houston Street, a few seconds before the shots were fired. Just prior to the shooting, David F. Powers, riding the Secret Service followup car, remarked to Kenneth O'Donnell that it was 12:30 p.m., the time they were due at the Trade Mart. Seconds after the shooting, Roy Kellerman, riding in the front seat of the Presidential limousine, looked at his watch and said "12:30" to the driver, Special Agent Greer. The Dallas police radio log reflects that Chief of Police Curry reported the shooting of the President and issued his initial orders at 12:30 p.m.

Speed of the Limousine

William Greer, operator of the Presidential limousine, estimated the car's speed at the time of the first shot as 12 to 15 miles per hour. Other witnesses in the motorcade estimated the speed of the President's limousine from 7 to 22 miles per hour. A more precise determination has been made from motion pictures taken on the scene by an amateur photographer, Abraham Zapruder. Based on these films, the speed of the President's automobile is computed at an average speed of 11.2 miles per hour. The car maintained this average speed over a distance of approximately 136 feet immediately preceding the shot which struck the President in the head. While the car traveled this distance, the Zapruder camera ran 152 frames. Since the camera operates at a speed of 18.3 frames per second, it was calculated that the car required 8.3 seconds to cover the 136 feet. This represents a speed of 11.2 miles per hour.

In the Presidential Limousine

Mrs. John F. Kennedy, on the left of the rear seat of the limousine, looked toward her left and waved to the crowds along the route. Soon after the motorcade turned onto Elm Street, she heard a sound similar to a motorcycle noise and a cry from Governor Connally, which caused her to look to her right. On turning she saw a quizzical look on her husband's face as he raised his left hand to his throat. Mrs. Kennedy then heard a second shot and saw the President's skull torn open under the impact of the bullet. As she cradled her mortally wounded husband, Mrs. Kennedy cried, "Oh, my God, they have shot my husband. I love you, Jack."

Governor Connally testified that he recognized the first noise as a rifle shot and the thought immediately crossed his mind that it was an assassination attempt. From his position in the right jump seat immediately in front of the President, he instinctively turned to his right because the shot appeared to come from over his right shoulder. Unable to see the President as he turned to the right, the Governor started to look back over his left shoulder, but he never completed the turn because he felt something strike him in the back. In his testimony before the Commission, Governor Connally was certain that he was hit by the second shot, which he stated he did not hear.

Mrs. Connally, too, heard a frightening noise from her right. Looking over her right shoulder, she saw that the President had both hands at his neck but she observed no blood and heard nothing. She watched as he slumped down with an empty expression on his face. Roy Kellerman, in the right front seat of the limousine, heard a report like a firecracker pop. Turning to his right in the direction of the noise, Kellerman heard the President say "My God, I am hit,"* and saw both the President's hands move up toward his neck. As he told the driver, "Let's get out of here; we are hit," Kellerman grabbed his microphone and radioed ahead to the lead car, "We are hit. Get us to the hospital immediately."

The driver, William Greer, heard a noise which he took to be a backfire from one of the motorcycles flanking the Presidential car. When he heard the same noise again, Greer glanced over his shoulder and saw Governor Connally fall. At the sound of the second shot he realized that something was wrong, and he pressed down on the accelerator as Kellerman said, "Get out of here fast." As he issued his instructions to Greer and to the lead car, Kellerman heard a "flurry of shots" within 5 seconds of the first noise. According to Kellerman, Mrs. Kennedy then cried out: "What are they doing to you?" Looking back from the front seat, Kellerman saw Governor Connally in his wife's lap and Special Agent Clinton J. Hill

---

*Kellerman is in error. The condition of the trachea after the nonfatal shot made it impossible for the President to utter distinguishable words and phrases. (C.G.W.)

lying across the trunk of the car.

Mrs. Connally heard a second shot fired and pulled her husband down into her lap. Observing his blood-covered chest as he was pulled into his wife's lap, Governor Connally believed himself mortally wounded. He cried out, "Oh, no, no, no. My God, they are going to kill us all." At first Mrs. Connally thought that her husband had been killed, but then she noticed an almost imperceptible movement and knew that he was still alive. She said, "It's all right. Be still." The Governor was lying with his head on his wife's lap when he heard a shot hit the President. At that point, both Governor and Mrs. Connally observed brain tissue splattered over the interior of the car. According to Governor and Mrs. Connally, it was after this shot that Kellerman issued his emergency instructions and the car accelerated.

Reaction by Secret Service Agents

From the left front running board of the President's followup car, Special Agent Hill was scanning the few people standing on the south side of Elm Street after the motorcade had turned off Houston Street. He estimated that the motorcade had slowed down to approximately 9 or 10 miles per hour on the turn at the intersection of Houston and Elm Streets and then proceeded at a rate of 12 to 15 miles per hour with the followup car trailing the President's automobile by approximately 5 feet. Hill heard a noise, which seemed to be a firecracker, coming from his right rear. He immediately looked to his right, "and in so doing, my eyes had to cross the Presidential limousine and I saw President Kennedy grab at himself and lurch forward and to the left." Hill jumped from the followup car and ran to the President's automobile. At about the time he reached the President's automobile, Hill heard a second shot, approximately 5 seconds after the first, which removed a portion of the President's head.

At the instant Hill stepped onto the left rear step of the President's automobile and grasped the handhold, the car lurched forward, causing him to lose his footing. He ran three or four steps, regained his position, and mounted the car. Between the time he originally seized the handhold and the time he mounted the car, Hill recalled that —

Mrs. Kennedy had jumped up from the seat and was, it appeared to me, reaching for something coming off the right rear bumper of the car, the right rear tail, when she noticed that I was trying to climb on the car. She turned toward me and I grabbed her and put her back in the back seat, crawled up on top of the back seat and lay there.

David Powers, who witnessed the scene from the President's followup car, stated that Mrs. Kennedy would probably have fallen off the rear end of the car and been killed if Hill had not pushed her back into the Presidential automobile. Mrs. Kennedy had no recollection of climbing onto the back of the car.

Special Agent Ready, on the right front running board of the Presidential followup car, heard noises that sounded like firecrackers and ran toward the President's limousine. But he was immediately called back by Special Agent Emory P. Roberts, in charge of the followup car, who did not believe that he could reach the President's car at the speed it was then traveling. Special Agent George W. Hickey, Jr., in the rear seat of the Presidential followup car, picked up and cocked an automatic rifle as he heard the last shot. At this point the cars were speeding through the underpass and had left the scene of the shooting, but Hickey kept the automatic weapon ready as the car raced to the hospital. Most of the other Secret Service agents in the motorcade had drawn their sidearms. Roberts noticed that the Vice President's car was approximately one-half block behind the Presidential followup car at the time of the shooting and signaled for it to move in closer.

Directing the security detail for the Vice President from the right front seat of the Vice-Presidential car, Special Agent Youngblood recalled:

As we were beginning to go down this incline, all of a sudden there was an explosive noise. I quickly observed unnatural movement of crowds, like ducking or scattering, and quick movements in the Presidential followup car. So I turned around and hit the Vice President on the shoulder and hollered, get down, and then looked around again and saw more of this movement, and so I proceeded to go to the back seat and get on top of him.

Youngblood was not positive that he was in the rear seat

before the second shot, but thought it probable because of President Johnson's statement to the effect immediately after the assassination. President Johnson emphasized Young-blood's instantaneous reaction after the first shot:

> I was startled by the sharp report or explosion, but I had no time to speculate as to its origin because Agent Young-blood turned in a flash, immediately after the first explo-sion, hitting me on the shoulder, and shouted to all of us in the back seat to get down. I was pushed down by Agent Youngblood. Almost in the same moment in which he hit or pushed me, he vaulted over the back seat and sat on me. I was bent over under the weight of Agent Youngblood's body, toward Mrs. Johnson and Senator Yarborough.

Clifton C. Carter, riding in the Vice President's followup car a short distance behind, reported that Youngblood was in the rear seat using his body to shield the Vice President before the second and third shots were fired.

Other Secret Service agents assigned to the motorcade re-mained at their posts during the race to the hospital. None stayed at the scene of the shooting, and none entered the Texas School Book Depository Building at or immediately after the shooting. Secret Service procedure requires that each agent stay with the person being protected and not be diverted unless it is necessary to accomplish the protective assignment. Forrest V. Sorrels, special agent in charge of the Dallas office, was the first Secret Service agent to return to the scene of the assassination, approximately 20 to 25 minutes after the shots were fired.

Distance of the Shots

According to the Commission's reconstruction, the President was a little over 88 yards from the rifle, if it were in the sixth floor window of the Texas School Book Depository; the angle downward from the rifle to the head is stated to be 15 degrees, 21 minutes (Report, p. 110).

> By using the Zapruder, Nix, and Muchmore motion pic-tures, the President's location at the time the bullet penetrated his head was fixed with reasonable precision. A careful anal-ysis of the Nix and Muchmore films led to fixing the exact

location of these cameramen. The point of impact of the bullet on the President's head was apparent in all of the movies. At that point in the Nix film a straight line was plotted from the camera position to a fixed point in the background and the President's location along this line was marked on a plat map. A similar process was followed with the Muchmore film. The President's location on that plat map was identical to that determined from the Nix film. The President's location, established through the Nix and Muchmore films, was confirmed by comparing his position on the Zapruder film. This location had hitherto only been approximated, since there were no landmarks in the background of the Zapruder frame for alinement purposes other than a portion of a painted line on the curb. Through these procedures, it was determined that President Kennedy was shot in the head when he was 230.8 feet from the point on the west curbline on Houston Street where it intersected with Elm Street. The President was 265.3 feet from the rifle in the sixth-floor window and at that position the approximate angle of declination was 15°21'.

Other Reports

The *Facts on File* (1963) described the details of the assassination shortly after the incident occurred. The presidential parade began at Love Field in Dallas, Texas. President and Mrs. Kennedy and Governor and Mrs. Connally were in the special presidential limousine. The protective "bubble top" was down. President Kennedy was scheduled to speak later in Dallas at the Trade Mart. The crowd along the parade route was enthusiastically friendly. Immediately behind the presidential limousine was a sedan with Secret Service men riding in it. Behind that Secret Service car another open-topped convertible carried Vice-president and Mrs. Johnson, along with Senator Yarborough of Texas. According to *Facts on File* (1963), as the car containing the President approached an underpass which led into Stemmons Freeway, three shots rang out. The report said, "The first two bullets hit the President who was sitting with Mrs. Kennedy in the rear seat, and he fell face down on the seat." The report continued and asserted clearly that a third bullet hit Governor Connally causing severe injuries, but which were not fatal. "The bullet tore through Connally's back, smashed three ribs, punctured his lung, broke his wrist, and penetrated his left thigh." The story went on to say that all the shots came from a window on the sixth floor of the Texas School Book Depository Building. According to that contemporary story, President Kennedy lost consciousness as soon as he was hit in the head by one of the bullets. At no time after that did he regain consciousness.

The Chief Surgeon of Parkland Memorial Hospital, Doctor Tom Shires, who was also Professor of Surgery at the University of Texas, Southwest Medical School, maintained that President Kennedy never knew what hit him. The precise time biologically that the President died is, of course, not known. Officially the death is listed as having occurred at 1:00 PM Dallas time. Doctor Shires further admitted that the President was biologically dead when he was brought into the hospital. Heroic attempts at resuscitation resulted in a feeble suggestion of a heartbeat.

The point to be remembered here is that, in a contemporary news story written while the events were clearly in mind and not confused by the legalistic maneuverings of lawyers conducting Hearings, it is clear that three shots in fact were fired on that horrible day. Two of the shots struck the President and a separate and distinct bullet wounded Governor Connally seriously but not fatally. With the passage of time and because of individual interests that somehow or another seemed to require being served, some rather strange theories were proposed in an attempt to suggest, as the Warren Commission finally did, that a single bullet, in fact, inflicted the nonfatal wounds on Kennedy and on Governor Connally respectively (*Facts on File,* 1963).

Contemporary Scene

In the Britannica *Book of the Year for 1964,* page 628, there is a picture of the late President Kennedy in the official presidential limousine. The caption under the picture asserts that the picture was taken "moments before the shooting." The source of the picture is obscure. Encyclopeadia Britannica business files do not go back that far. In the picture, the late President, moments before the shooting, has his right arm resting on the rim of the limousine body adjacent to him. His hand is raised to about midchest level. His suit coat on the right side is hitched upward to a minimal rounded fold toward his head. What is visible of his shirt suggests no such upward folding.

There is then the possibility that the suit coat may have been folded upward and that the resulting entrance hold in the coat is in fact lower than it might ordinarily be if the coat were smooth over the shoulders of the victim. However, the shirt shows no such upward folding. It therefore seems probable that the location of the hole in the President's shirt gives a fairly good indication of the level of the entrance hole of the bullet which struck the President in the back.

No mention in the Warren Report is made of the late President's undershirt. Was he wearing any? What happened to the body brace? Do either of these items, if in existence, show bullet holes? Where?

The Value of Motion Pictures of the Event

Abraham Zapruder will go down in history as the amateur photographer whose color motion picture film was used extensively to calibrate the events of the assassination. The Warren Commission was hypnotized by the film, as apparently the FBI and, subsequent to the publishing of the Report, a host of critics and defenders of the Report also were.

As Milton Helpern pointed out, "Even those who have purported to study the work of the Commission in considered hindsight are mesmerized by the beguiling and misleading power of the Zapruder movie" (Houts, 1967).

Arlen Specter, a lawyer with the Commission staff, used the film to time events not in the film itself but at a point at least thirty yards away, in the Texas School Book Depository Building. Helpern has emphasized that the film, whether run forward or backward, tells nothing about the timing of any events in the assassination. The reason is simple; there is nothing in the motion picture itself to serve as a precise measurement of any event. The contention that the President or Connally "reacted" visibly to a given wound at the precise instant that it occurred is biologically unsound. What is known about the biological responses to gunshot wounds is that such instantaneous reaction occurs rarely; as a supposition in the Kennedy murder it is of no value.

There is no yardstick in the Zapruder film that permits investigators to use it as the basic time reference for the course of events in the murder scene. Such use has been and continues to be misleading.

The Press Conferences

The doctors who treated the late President at Parkland Memorial Hospital were forced into a number of press conferences at which they answered questions about their first hand observations of the wounds and the cause of death.

Some news reports suggested that the President had been shot in the front of the head or in the right temple. Doctor Perry was reported to have said over radio station WOR on 22 November 1963 at about 1443 hours CST that an entrance wound was seen in the front of the President's head.

Chet Huntley on NBC News at 1347 hours CST reported that Kennedy had been shot in the right temple. Admiral Burkley, the President's personal physician, apparently at that time agreed with the report and volunteered that it was a simple matter of a bullet going through the President's head.

Later during the day of the murder, Doctor Perry was reported by the Associated Press as admitting that the President was shot in the front of the head. The NBC log of 22 November 1963, page 8, listed a report quoting Doctor Perry and Doctor Clark as agreeing that the President was shot "in front as he faced the assailant"; the listed time was 1436 hours CST.

A problem with these news reports is that the Secret Service failed to supply to the Warren Commission recordings of the various press conferences. Apparently some representative of the Secret Service had promised that such recordings would be obtained and made available. The National Archives has yet to admit the existence of any such recordings in the files of the Warren Commission.

Later during sworn testimony before the Commission, the Parkland doctors who had taken part, quite legally, in various press conferences were subjected to innuendo and the questioning was so threatening as to make several of them play down what they had said and indeed to claim that the confusion of the time had made their comments misunderstood by the reporters.

CHAPTER 4

MEDICAL TREATMENT OF THE VICTIMS

THE scene at Parkland Hospital after the shooting of President Kennedy was chaotic. Medical personnel and support personnel came from various parts of the hospital, and at the same time a throng of presidential advisors, hangers-on, and police personnel milled around the vicinity of the emergency room.

According to Doctor Charles J. Carrico, a surgical resident at Parkland Memorial Hospital, President Kennedy, upon arrival in the emergency room, showed slow respiration that was spasmodic; Doctor Carrico described it as agonal (Hearings, vol. 6, pp. 1-7). Carrico was the first doctor to reach the President upon his arrival at the hospital. He was described as cyanotic and as showing no spontaneous movements. "We opened his shirt and coat and tie and observed the small wound in the anterior lower third of the neck." No sucking wounds of the chest were observed. There was a large skull and scalp wound recognized. "There seemed to be a 4 to 5 cm area of avulsion of the scalp and the skull was fragmented and bleeding cerebral and cerebellar tissue" [sic]. For reference, 5 cm is about 2 inches; 4 cm is about 1.6 inch.

Doctor Carrico described the anterior neck wound as 4 to 7 mm in diameter, almost in the midline but slightly to the right ("maybe a little to the right of the midline"). Was that location given as viewed from the front or in terms of the President's right and left sides? The hole was round and showed no ragged edges or "stellate lacerations."

Carrico was of the opinion that the cause of death was "a head injury."

A hypothetical question given him by Arlen Specter was phrased to lead to agreement that the hole in the neck could have been an entrance or an exit wound.

Doctor Malcolm O. Perry, Assistant Professor of Surgery at

Southwestern Medical School of the University of Texas, also testified to his activities in the Parkland Memorial Hospital emergency room.

When he entered the room, he described what he saw. "I noted there was a large wound of the right posterior parietal area in the head exposing lacerated brain. There was blood and brain tissue on the cart. The President's eyes were deviated and dilated and he was unresponsive. There was a small wound in the lower anterior third in the midline of the neck, from which blood was exuding very slowly."

Perry described the neck wound as "spherical" (circular? round?) to oval in shape. It was not a ragged wound nor did it have a punched-out appearance; it was a clean-cut wound about 5 mm in diameter.

In order to insert a tube into the President's windpipe more adequately, Doctor Perry made a transverse incision from right to left through the existing hole in the throat. He then observed, "There was an injury to the right lateral aspect of the trachea at the level of the external wound. The trachea was deviated slightly to the left and it was necessary to divide the strap muscles on the left side in order to gain access to the trachea" (Hearings, vol. 6, pp. 7-18).

After that, the wound in the trachea was enlarged surgically to admit the tracheotomy tube.

It is also important in the light of the later autopsy report to recognize that Doctor Perry, a certified surgeon, said, "The pressure of this free blood and air in this area (the superior right mediastinum) could be indicative of a wound of the right hemithorax, and I asked that someone put a right chest tube in for seal drainage." This was done by two other surgeons, Doctor Baxter and Doctor Peters.

Doctor Perry testified that he did not have adequate information to conclude whether the throat wound was an entrance or an exit nor anything about the trajectory of the bullet.

The questioning of Doctor Perry by Arlen Specter was peculiar. There was an accusatory air about it as if Perry were guilty of something or other. It was a cross-examination type of exercise in which Specter seemed to be trying to impeach

Doctor Perry for some kind of behavior or some sort of statement that he may have made.

Perry agreed that the cause of death was "massive brain trauma with attendant severe hemorrhage."

In the questioning by Specter, it is obvious that Doctor Perry was being browbeaten in order to have him testify that he knew nothing about the direction or trajectory of the bullet or bullets. He was faced with what Specter called "facts" about the trajectory and questioned in such an accusatory way that he could only answer that the throat wound he saw was "compatible" with the assertions in Specter's imaginative, hypothetical question; "compatible" is, of course, a meaningless term often used by lawyers and doctors to obfuscate rather than to inform.

Medical Treatment

The doctors and administrators at Parkland Memorial Hospital, where the President breathed his last, were understandably concerned that there would be no adverse criticism of the manner in which they treated the moribund President from the medical point of view. Needless to say, the facts clearly demonstrate that all the appropriate medical procedures for that particular patient were carried out quickly and with skill.

In Commission Exhibit Number 392, there is a series of reports by medical personnel who first saw the wounded Kennedy and ministered to his needs.* These reports were filed by

---

*Commission Exhibit Number 392 as it appears in Appendix VIII of the Report is peculiar. The first page of the exhibit (p. 516 of the Report) is a short piece of what seems to be a sliced-off portion of a larger sheet of paper. In the upper right hand corner is the handwritten word "statement." Centered at the top border of the partial sheet is a paste-on label reading "Commission Exhibit No. 392." The typing on that sheet and the form of the typing differ markedly from the rest of the exhibit, which continues with "Summary" on page 517 of the Report. No explanation is given for the strange arrangement. In addition, the quality of reproduction of the handwritten statements of the various doctors from Parkland Hospital varies for no apparent reason: On page 523 of the Report, Doctor Baxter's statement is reproduced sharply; on the next two pages, the statement of Doctor Clark is so badly done as to be almost illegible; finally on page 526, the first part of Doctor McClelland's statement is clear and sharp while the last few lines and his signature reproduced on page 527 are of poor quality. This sort of poor quality control is quite uncharacteristic of the Government Printing Office under usual conditions.

skilled, certified specialists in the medical profession. Because of the types of cases that were common in the emergency room of Parkland Hospital, these doctors were familiar with gunshot wounds.

As part of the Exhibit Number 392, the Director of Neurological Surgery, Parkland Hospital, Doctor Kemp Clark reported the President's wounds as he saw them firsthand shortly after the shooting. "Two external wounds, one in the lower third of the anterior neck, the other in the occipital region of the skull, were noted. Through the head wound, blood and brain were extruding. Dr. Carrico inserted a cuffed endotracheal tube. While doing so, he noted a ragged wound of the trachea immediately below the larynx."

He continued, "There was a large wound in the right occipito-parietal region, from which profuse bleeding was occurring. 1500 cc. of blood were estimated on the drapes and floor of the Emergency Operating Room. There was considerable loss of scalp and bone tissue. Both cerebral and cerebellar tissue was extruding from the wound."

Doctor Perry reported that a tracheotomy was performed. While performing the manipulation, "a right lateral injury to the trachea was noted."

Doctor Robert N. McClelland wrote his admission note about the President on 22 November 1963, at 4:45 PM while all the facts were still vivid in his mind. The President was reported dead at 1300 hours that day (1:00 PM). Several of Doctor McClelland's observations recorded while they were still fresh in his memory are of interest. "The President was at that time comatose from a massive gunshot wound of the head with a fragment wound of the trachea." McClelland's report, which is part of Commission Exhibit Number 392, concludes, "The cause of death was due to massive head and brain injury from a gunshot wound of the left temple." Doctor McClelland was in a position at the treatment table to get a clear view of the President's head.

In the turmoil of that day, it could be that a qualified surgeon would get left confused with right; it is vaguely possible that he might get the temporal region mixed up with the parietal or occipital. The probability of such confusion is rather low however. Adequate clarification of the gunshot wound of the "left temple" did not develop during or after the Warren Commission Hearings.

With respect to the reported wound in the left temple of the President's body, Doctor McClelland on 21 March 1964 gave a deposition to the Commission concerning his report of the wound (Commission Exhibit No. 392). He was asked under oath by Specter "whether in fact you did make this report and submit it to the authorities at Parkland Hospital?" McClelland's answer was an unequivocal yes. He was further asked by Specter, "And are all the facts set forth true and correct to the best of your knowledge, information and belief?"

McClelland responded, "To the best of my knowledge, yes."

On 21 March 1964 Specter took a deposition from another Parkland Hospital doctor, Kemp Clark, who admitted that he had not seen a wound in the left temple of the President's body. He was not familiar with Doctor McClelland's observation and could not account for the origin of the report.

Doctor Marion Jenkins, also of Parkland Hospital, questioned by Specter on that same day in March, clearly stated, "I don't know whether this is right or not, but I thought there was a wound on the left temporal area, right at the hairline and right above the zygomatic process."

When Specter claimed that the autopsy report showed no such wound, Jenkins responded in an obviously troubled way. He had observed the pneumothorax during treatment of the dying President and obviously wondered about the "intact" pleural lining of the chest cavity reported by the pathologists. The absence of any report at autopsy of a wound in the left temple also seemed to leave him uneasy; he and another attending surgeon had gained the impression of such a wound during their contact with the dying President.

Moreover, in the *Philadelphia Sunday Bulletin* for 24 November 1963 Father Oscar Huber, who gave the Last Rites to President Kennedy, was reported to have observed a terrible wound over the left eye of the President.

Doctor Adolph Giesecke responded during his testimony to

Specter on 25 March 1964 concerning the left head wound. "It seemed that from the vertex to the left ear, and from the browline to the occiput on the left-hand side of the head the cranium was entirely missing." When queried specifically about the side of the head where the wound was, Doctor Giesecke repeated that as far as he could remember it was the left side of the head.

There is also a 0.4 cm hole, particle, or some defect marked at the left eye on the autopsy sheet prepared at the table by Doctor Thornton Boswell (Commission Exhibit No. 397).

When these data are put together, they suggest that adequate reason existed for the Commission to demand a thorough and detailed study of the autopsy photographs and x-rays to clarify just what damage had occurred to the left side of the head. Wounds in that region of the body would be crucial to an adequate medicolegal interpretation of the entire case. The fact that the Commission and its staff let the matter rest suggests gross incompetence or deliberate neglect of obviously important information in the case.

Autopsy v. Clinical Record

There is some confusion in the autopsy as compared with the clinical record from Parkland Hospital concerning the condition of the chest cavity of the President. In the official summary of the medical treatment given to the President and signed by Kemp Clark, M.D., Director, Service of Neurological Surgery, it was stated that Doctor Robert McClelland, attending surgeon, arrived to help in the President's care. Doctors Perry, Baxter, and McClelland began a tracheotomy, as considerable quantities of blood were present from the President's oropharynx. At this time, Doctor Paul Peters, attending Neurological Surgeon, and Doctor Kemp Clark arrived. Because of the lacerated trachea, anterior chest tubes were placed in both pleural spaces. These were connected to sealed underwater drainage.

During Doctor Humes testimony about the autopsy (Hearings, vol. 2, p. 363), he said, "we then opened his chest cavity, and we very carefully examined the lining of his chest cavity and both of his lungs. We found that there was, in fact, no defect in the pleural lining of the President's chest. It was completely intact." Here there is confusion with respect to the report from Parkland Memorial Hospital and the report from the autopsy. The clinical report said that incisions were made into the chest on either side and drainage tubes were placed in the pleural cavity. The autopsy report described the location of these knife wounds, as they are called. However, it was claimed by Doctor Humes that these cuts went only through the skin and did not actually enter the chest cavity. This confusion in what actually occurred is extremely common concerning all of the medicolegal aspects of President Kennedy's murder.

Further, on the Parkland Memorial Hospital admission note signed by Malcom O. Perry, M.D., 1630 hours, 22 November 1963 it was stated that a tracheotomy tube was put in place and the cuff inflated and respiration assisted. Closed chest cardiac massage was initiated after placement of sealed-drainage chest tubes, but without benefit. So again the mention of tubes into the chest of the dying President was claimed. On the other hand, the autopsy report of the chest cavity claimed it to be intact. Nowhere since that time has there been an explanation to bring together in some understandable manner these conflicting reports.

Surgeon Charles Baxter, M.D., on a Parkland Memorial Hospital admission note concerning President Kennedy's assassination, said that when he arrived at the emergency room a left chest tube was being inserted and a cutdown was being made on the left arm. The President was obviously moribund, there was no pulse as far as he could determine. Then Doctors Perry and Baxter inserted a right chest drainage tube in the second intercostal space anteriorly in the chest. Again, two competent and recognized surgeons maintained that in the anterior chest wall there were two drainage tubes inserted into the chest cavity.

According to Doctor McClelland of the Parkland Memorial Hospital, he was also called to the emergency room. The tracheotomy was performed by Doctor Perry, Doctor Baxter, and Doctor McClelland. This procedure was done to relieve respiratory distress. Then two other physicians, Doctor Jones and Doctor Peters, according to Doctor McClelland, inserted bilateral anterior chest tubes for relief of the chest condition attendent upon the injury to the tracheal region. Another statement comes from Doctor M.T. Jenkins, Professor and Chairman of the Department of Anesthesiology, University of Texas, Southwestern Medical School, who stated that at the same time in the emergency room, "Drs. Charles Baxter, Malcom Perry, and Robert McClelland arrived at the same time and began a tracheotomy and started the insertion of a right chest tube, since there was also obvious tracheal and chest damage. Drs. Paul Peters and Kemp Clark arrived simultaneously and immediately thereafter assisted respectively with the insertion of the right chest tube and with manual closed chest cardiac compression to insure circulation."

A respectable battery of surgeons all maintained that chest drainage tubes were inserted into the President's body. The autopsy reported only a completely intact pleural cavity. There is no way at the moment to decide who was correct, who was misinformed, or who had a lapse of memory. The fact remains that, in a situation like this, if observations at autopsy are open to question, where else in the overall pathological examination of the President are there similar examples of questionable procedure and questionable remembrances?

This question becomes more critical when it is realized that the basic information presented to the Commission and accepted by the Commission on the wounds of the President was not basic at all.

Doctor McClelland described an anterior neck wound as told to him by Doctor Perry. "it was a very small injury, with clean-cut, although somewhat irregular margins of less than a quarter inch in diameter, with minimal tissue damage surrounding it on the skin" (Hearings, vol. 6, pp. 32-33).

After an accusatory type of interchange with Arlen Specter, Doctor McClelland continued to maintain that "if I were simply looking at the wound again and had seen the wound in its unchanged state . . . if I saw the wound in its state in which Dr. Perry described it to me, I would .. think this were an entrance wound ... not knowing anything more than just seeing the wound itself" (Hearings, vol. 6, p. 37).

Doctor Carrico, in answer to a question from attorney Specter about the anterior throat wound, said, "This was probably a 4-7 mm. wound, almost in the midline, maybe a little to the right of the midline, and below the thyroid cartilage. It was, as I recall, rather round and there were no jagged edges or stellate lacerations" (Hearings, vol. 6, p. 3).

It is obvious that Doctor Carrico, a trained surgeon, was describing an entrance wound and certainly not an exit wound made by a military bullet. At that time, Doctor Carrico had observed in his practice of medicine nearly two hundred gunshot wounds.

Doctor Baxter maintained that it was unlikely that the throat wound could have been an exit wound (Hearings, vol. 6, p. 42). He had observed at that time about five hundred gunshot wounds per year for a period of six years.

Doctor Jones evaluated the anterior throat wound as a bullet wound of entrance; he was not forced out of that opinion by pressure of the interrogating attorney (Hearings, vol. 6, p. 55). Jones was familiar with as many as four to five gunshot wounds per night for long periods of time.

Doctor Akin, an anesthesiologist, observed the anterior throat wound which he placed below the level of the cricoid cartilage. He was unequivocal in interpreting it to be an entrance wound.

As an interesting aside, Arlen Specter asked each doctor from Parkland Memorial Hospital whether he had had special training in gunshot wounds; the implication was that without such special training, testimony contrary to the already established conclusions of the Commission would have little weight. A similar question might be asked of Specter; what "special" training did he have in gunshot wounds, ballistic science, and pathology that would permit him to formulate a theory of wounding involving complex considerations of a highly technical nature? When he did so theorize, should the result be given any serious consideration, based on the competence of the theorizer?

Doctor Perry, who performed the tracheotomy that modified

the anterior throat wound, made it clear that he had cut *across* the lower part of the hole to enlarge it; he had not cut out the hole as the Report of the Commission implied. Thus, at autopsy the cut edges could have been realigned and the hole of controversy approximately reconstructed. Doctor Perry also saw free air and blood in the superior right mediastinum; this observation was strong evidence that there was a wound of the right hemithorax. For that reason, chest tubes were inserted into the thoracic cavity. The invasion of the cavity was not found by the autopsy team.

Doctor M.T. Jenkins, Professor and Chairman, Department of Anesthesiology, Southwestern Medical School, summarized the President's head wound in a memo to the Parkland Hospital Administrator, C.J. Price (Commission Exhibit No. 392) as follows. "There was a great laceration of the right side of the head (temporal and occipital), causing a great defect in the skull plate so that there was herniation and laceration of great areas of the brain, even to the extent that the cerebellum had protruded from the wound. There were also fragmented sections of brain on the drapes of the emergency room cart. With the institution of adequate cardiac compression, there was a great flow of blood from the cranial cavity, indicating that there was much vascular damage as well as brain tissue damage."

It is clear that the damage to the head structures from the bullet or bullets was extensive and massive. The cerebellum lies deep at the base of the brain. The fact that it protruded from the wound strongly suggests that a hunting-style bullet may well have struck the President's head.

GOVERNOR CONNALLY

Governor Connally received serious wounds from a bullet. He underwent surgery at the hospital, and subsequently, made a full recovery.

From the first the Governor maintained that Kennedy was struck by the first shot but that he was wounded by a separate and distinct second shot (Fig. 4-1).

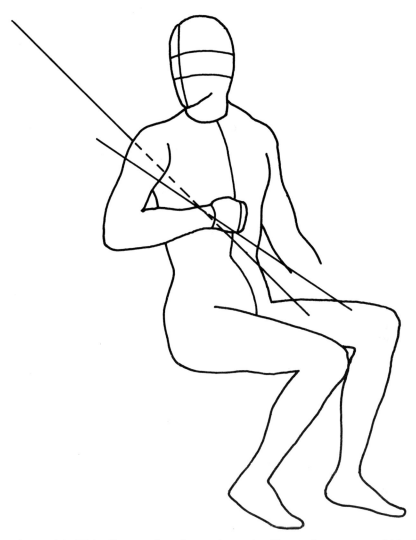

Figure 4-1. This diagram is redrawn from the illustration on page 346 of volume 17, Exhibits. It is Commission Exhibit Number 689. It shows in the Commission's words, "Diagram of body in sitting position, marked by Dr. Shaw, to show position of Governor Connally at time of the assassination and inclination of bullet to cause all three wounds." The downward angle of the bullet is so steep as to make it improbable that the bullet said to have gone through Kennedy nonfatally was the same bullet that went through Connally. The lateral entry of this bullet into the *extreme* right side of Connally's chest demanded that a single bullet make two right-angle turns in midair in order to get to the entry locus in Connally after going through Kennedy. This diagram is strong evidence that at least two shooters were involved.

In the Report (p. 92) it is stated that the surgeon who was involved in the successful treatment of Connally, Doctor Robert Shaw, concluded that the wound in the extreme right back of the Governor was an entry wound because "of the small size and clean-cut edges."

Strangely, later in the Report (p. 109), that small bullet hole in the back is described as "the large wound" which is said to result from a yawing bullet or a tangential strike (Hearings, vol. 6, p. 95).

Shaw concluded that the hole in Connally's anterior chest was an exit; it was a two-inch opening with ragged edges (Report, p. 92).

The size of the wound in Connally's back is not certain. In Commission Exhibit Number 392, it is reported by Doctor Shaw to be 1.2 inches in greatest diameter. In the Hearings he states that the longest diameter of the back wound was 0.6 inch (Hearings, vol. 6, p. 85; vol. 4, p. 104).

The bullet hole that remained in the Governor's suit coat, after the coat had been inexplicably dry cleaned and pressed before it was studied, measured about 0.25 by 0.65 inch. That size is compatible with the smaller size of the back wound.

Furthermore, "Dr. Shaw measured with a caliper an angle of declination of 25° from the point of entry on the back to the point of exit on the front of the Governor's chest" (Report, p. 93).

The following reports are taken verbatim from Commission Exhibit Number 392 and summarize the surgical treatment given the wounded Governor at Parkland Memorial Hospital.

> The patient was brought to the OR from the EOR. In the EOR a sucking wound of the right chest was partially controlled by occlusive dressing supported by manual pressure. A tube had been placed through the second interspace in the mid-clavicular line connected to a waterseal bottle to evacuate the right pneumothorax and hemathorax. An IV infusion of RL solution had already been started. As soon as the patient was positioned on the OR table, the anesthesia, was induced by Dr. Giesecke and an endotracheal tube was in place. As soon as it was possible to control respiration with positive pressure the occlusive dressing was taken from the right chest

and the extent of the wound more carefully determined. It was found that the wound of entrance was just lateral to the right scapula close to the axilla, yet had passed through the latysmus [*sic*] dorsi muscle, shattered approximately ten cm of the lateral and anterior portion of the right fifth rib, and emerged below the right nipple. The wound of entrance was approximately three cm in its longest diameter and the wound of exit was a ragged wound approximately 5 cm in its greatest diameter. The skin and subcutaneous tissue over the path of the missile moved in a paradoxical manner with respiration indicating softening of the chest. The skin of the whole area was carefully cleansed with Phisohex® and Iodine. The entire area including the wound entrance and wound of exit was draped partially excluding the wound of entrance for the first part of the operation. An elliptical incision was made around the wound of exit removing the torn edges of the skin and the damaged subcutaneous tissue. The incision was then carried in a downward curve up toward the right axilla so as to not have the skin incision over the actual path of the missile through the chest wall. This incision was carried down through the subcutaneous tissue to expose the Serratus anterior muscle and the anterior border of the lattissimus dorsi muscle. The fragmented and damaged portions of the Serratus anterior muscle were excised. Small rib fragments that were adhering to periosteal tags were carefully removed preserving as much periosteum as possible. The fourth intercostal muscle bundle and fifth intercostal muscle bundle were not appreciably damaged. The ragged ends of the damaged fifth rib were cleaned out with the rongeur. The plura had been torn open by the secondary missiles created by the fragmented fifth rib. The wound was open widely and exposure was obtained with a self retaining retractor. The right pleural cavity was then carefully inspected. Approximately 200 cc of clot and liquid blood was removed from the pleural cavity. The middle lobe had a linear rent starting at its peripheral edge going down towards its hilum separating the lobe into two segments. There was an open bronchus in the depth of this wound. Since the vascularity and the bronchial connections to the lobe were intact, it was decided to repair the lobe rather than to remove it. The repair was accomplished with a running suture of #000 chromic gut on a traumatic needle closing both plural surfaces as well as two running sutures approximating the tissue of the central portion of the lobe. This almost completely sealed off the air leaks which were evident in the torn portion of the lobe. The lower lobe was next examined and found to be engorged with blood and at one point a laceration allowed the oozing of blood. This laceration had undoubtedly been caused by a rib fragment. This laceration was closed with a single suture of #3-0 chromic gut on a traumatic needle. The right pleural cavity was not carefully examined and small ribs fragments were removed, the diaphram was found to be uninjured. There was no evidence of injury of the mediastinum and its contents. Hemostasis had been accomplished within the pleural cavity with the repair of the middle lobe and the suturing of the laceration of the lower lobe. The upper lobe was found to be uninjured. The drains which had previously been placed in the second interspace in the midclavicular line was found to be longer than necessary so approximately ten cm of it was cut away and the remaining portion was tenonstrated with two additional openings. An additional drain was placed through a stab wound in the eighth interspace in the posterior axillary line. Both these drains were then connected to a waterseal bottle. The fourth and fifth intercostal muscles were then approximated with interrupted sutures of #0 chromic gut. The remaining portion of the Serratus anterior muscle was then approximated across the closure of the intercostal muscle. The laceration of the latissimus dorsi muscle on its intermost surface was then closed with several interrupted sutures of #0 chromic gut. Before the closing the subcutaneous tissue one million units of Penicillin and one gram of Streptomycin in 100 cc normal saline was instilled into the wound. The stab wound was then made in the most dependent portion of the wound coming out near the angle of the scapula. A large Penrose drain was drawn out through this stab wound to allow drainage of the wound of the chest wall. The subcutaneous tissue was then closed with interrupted #0 chromic gut inverting the knots. Skin closed with interrupted certical mattress sutures of black silk. Attention was next turned to the wound of entrance. It was excised with an elliptical incision. It was found that the latissimus dorsi muscle although lacerated was not badly damaged so that the opening was closed with sutures of #0 chromic gut in the fascia of the muscle. Before closing this incision palpation with the index finger Penrose drain could be felt immediately below in the space beneath the latissimus dorsi muscle. The skin closed with interrupted vertical mattress sutures of black silk. Drainage tubes were secured with safety pins and adhesive tape and dressings applied. As soon as the operation on the chest had been concluded Dr. Gregory and Dr. Shires started the surgery that was necessary for the wounds of the right wrist and left thigh.

/s/

RS:bl   Dr. Robert Shaw

*There was also a comminuted fracture of the right radius secondary to the same missile and in addition a small flesh wound of the left thigh. The operative notes concerning the management of the right arm and left thigh will be dictated by Dr. Charles Gregory and Dr. Tom Shires.

While still under general anesthesia and following a thoracotomy and repair of the chest injury by Dr. Robert Shaw, the right upper extremity was thoroughly prepped in the routine fashion after shaving. He was draped in the routine fashion using stockinette, the only addition was the use of a debridement pan. The wound of entry on the dorsal aspect of the right wrist over the junction of the distal fourth of the radius and shaft was approximately two cm in length and rather oblique with the loss of tissue with some considerable contusion at the margins of it. There was a wound of exit along the volar surface of the wrist about two cm above the flexion crease of the wrist and in the midline. The wound of entrance was carefully excised and developed through the muscles and tendons from the radial side of that bone to the bone itself where the fracture was encountered. It was noted that the tendon of the abductor palmaris longus or Ext. Pol. Briois also a partial transection of the superficial radial nerve was transected, only two small fragments of bone were removed, one approximately one cm in length and consisted of lateral cortex which lay free in the wound and had no soft tissue connections, another much smaller fragment perhaps 3 mm in length was subsequently removed. Small bits of metal were encountered at various levels throughout the wound and these were wherever they were identified and could be picked up were picked up and have been submitted to the

Pathology department for identification and examination. Throughout the wound and especially in the superficial layers and to some extent in the tendon and tendon sheaths on the radial side of the arm small fine bits of cloth consistant with fine bits of Mohair. It is our understanding that the patient was wearing a Mohair suit at the time of the injury and this accounts for the deposition of such organic material within the wound. After as careful and complete a debridement as could be carried out and with an apparent integrity of the flexor tendons and the median nerve in the volar side, and after thorough irrigation of the wound of exit on the volar surface of the wrist was closed primarily with wire sutures while the wound of entrance on the radial side of the forearm was only partially closed, being left open for the purpose of drainage should any make spontaneous appearance. This is because of the presence of Mohair and organic material deep into the wound which is prone to produce tissue reactions and to encourage infection and this precaution of not closing the wound was taken in correspondance with our experience in that regard.

In view of the urgency of the Governor's original chest injury it was impossible to definitely ascertain the status of the circulation and the nerve supply to the hand and wrist on the right side. Accordingly, it was determined as best we could at the time of operation and the radial artery was found to be intact and pulsating normally. The integrity of the median nerve and the ulnar nerve is not clearly established but it is presumed to be present. Following closure of the volar wound and partial closure of the radial wound, dry sterile dressings were applied and a long arm cast was then applied with skin tape traction, rubber band variety, attached to the thumb and index finger of the right hand. An attitude of flexon was created at the right elbow, and post operatively the limbus suspended from an overhead frame using tape traction. The post operative diagnosis for the right forearm remains the same and again I suggest that you incorporate this particular dictation together with other dictations which will be given to you by the surgeons concerned with this patient.

/s/

CG:bl   Charles Gregory, M.D.

There was a 1 cm. punctate missile wound over the juncture of the middle and lower third, medial aspect, of the left thigh. X-rays of the thigh and leg revealed a bullet fragment which was imbedded in the body of the femur in the distal third. The leg was prepared with Phisohex and I.O. Prep and was draped in the usual fashion. Following this the missile wound was excised and the bullet tract was explored. The missile wound was seen to course through the subcutaneous fat and into the vastus medialis. The necrotic fat and muscle were debrided down to the region of the femur. The direction of the missile wound was judged not to be in the course of the femoral vessel, since the wound was distal and anterior to Hunter's canal. Following complete debridement of the wound and irrigation with saline, the wound was felt to be adequately debrided enough so that three simple through-and-through, stainless steel Aloe #28 wire sutures were used encompassing the skin, subcutaneous tissue, and muscle fascia on both sides. Following this a sterile dressing was applied. The dorsalis pedis and posterior tibial pulses in both legs were quite good. The thoracic procedure had been completed at this time, the debridement of the compound fracture in the arm was still in progress at the time this soft tissue injury repair was completed.

/s/

Tom Shires, M.D.

Contradictions

Internal contradictions in the Warren Report make it difficult at times to be certain just what was being contended by the authors.

For example on page 92 of the Report it is stated that the wound in Connally's back was of "small size" and it showed "clean-cut edges." These characteristics persuaded the surgeon, Doctor Robert Shaw, that it was an entry wound.

But on page 109 of the Report, it is stated that "the large wound on the Governor's back" could be explained in part by a bullet that was wobbling as it entered.

On page 107 of the Report it is stated that experiments performed by Army ballistics experts using a simulation of the

Governor's chest showed that the bullet could have been tumbling as it left the anterior chest. On that same page it is asserted that the test bullet "displayed characteristics similar to the bullet found on Governor Connally's stretcher" (Exhibit Nos. 399, 853; Hearings, vol. 5, p. 80).

However, that test bullet did not go through a simulated wrist. A test bullet that did impact a cadaver's wrist showed pronounced flattening and deformation of the nose. In reality, the so-called ballistics tests done for the Commission demonstrated nothing. In any event, they were not crucial. Careful examination of the wounded bodies would give crucial information of what did in fact happen. Such examination of Connally's body clearly indicates that he was not struck by the same bullet that produced Kennedy's nonfatal wound.

In Commission Exhibit Number 392, the Governor's back wound was placed lateral to the right scapula but passed through the latissimus dorsi muscle. This entrance wound in the back was 3 cm in longest diameter, about 1.2 inches. The exit wound in the anterior chest was ragged and about 5 cm in longest diameter, about 2 inches. No information seems available about the shortest diameter. The hole in the Governor's left thigh was about 0.39 inch in diameter. The wrist wounds were as follows: entry on dorsum about 0.79 inch and oblique; exit along volar surface, no size given.

Summation

Reports from Parkland Memorial Hospital as filed by the only physicians who saw the unaltered, original wounds of the late President Kennedy and of Governor Connally indicate the following.

1. President Kennedy had in his anterior throat a small hole that appeared to doctors familiar with gunshot wounds to be the entry wound of a bullet.
2. President Kennedy had a massive destruction of the right side of his head as a result of a gunshot wound. He probably died instantly as a result of that wound.
3. Several expert surgeons on the hospital staff who were

located immediately adjacent to the moribund President described a bullet wound to the *left* temporal region at about the hairline.

4. Governor Connally was wounded by a bullet that entered the extreme right side of his back in the upper thorax region. It passed through his body at a downward angle of 25 degrees, smashing part of his fifth right rib, producing a comminuted fracture of the right wrist, and leaving a piece of metal in his left thigh bone.

5. No wound in the back of the President's body was observed by the Parkland Memorial Hospital physicians.

6. No bullets were found by hospital doctors. Fragments of metal and of textile were removed from some of Connally's wounds.

7. A death certificate of questionable legality was executed by one of the hospital doctors, Doctor Kemp Clark. Cause of death was given as gunshot wound to the head. No serious examination of the dead body was made before issuance of the death certificate. It is reasonable to conclude from the information available that the certificate was issued in order to circumvent the Texas laws that applied to the transportation of remains of homicide victims.

CHAPTER 5

THE AUTOPSY ON THE
PRESIDENT'S REMAINS

THE Warren Commission summarized the autopsy activities as follows (Report, pp. 59-60).

Given a choice between the National Naval Medical Center at Bethesda, Md., and the Army's Walter Reed Hospital, Mrs. Kennedy chose the hospital at Bethesda for the autopsy because the President had served in the Navy. Mrs. Kennedy and the Attorney General, with three Secret Service agents, accompanied President Kennedy's body on the 45-minute automobile trip from Andrews AFB to the hospital. On the 17th floor of the Hospital, Mrs. Kennedy and the Attorney General joined other members of the Kennedy family to await the conclusion of the autopsy. Mrs. Kennedy was guarded by Secret Service agents in quarters assigned to her in the naval hospital. The Secret Service established a communication system with the White House and screened all telephone calls and visitors.

The hospital received the President's body for autopsy at approximately 7:35 p.m. X-rays and photographs were taken preliminarily and the pathological examination began at about 8 p.m. The autopsy report noted that President Kennedy was 46 years of age, 72 1/2 inches tall, weighted 170 pounds, had blue eyes and reddish-brown hair. The body was muscular and well developed with no gross skeletal abnormalities except for those caused by the gunshot wounds. Under "Pathological Diagnosis" the cause of death was set forth as "Gunshot wound, head."

The autopsy examination revealed two wounds in the President's head. One wound, approximately one-fourth of an inch by five-eighths of an inch (6 by 15 millimeters), was located about an inch (2.5 centimeters) to the right and slightly above the large bony protrusion (external occipital protuberance) which juts out at the center of the lower part of the back of the skull. The second head wound measured approximately 5 inches (13 centimeters) in its greatest diameter, but it was difficult to measure accurately because multiple crisscross fractures radiated from the large defect. During the autopsy examination, Federal agents brought the surgeons three pieces of bone recovered from Elm Street and the Presidential automobile. When put together, these fragments accounted for approximately three-quarters of the missing portion of the skull. The surgeons observed, through X-ray analysis, 30 or 40 tiny dustlike fragments of metal running in a line from the wound in the rear of the President's head toward the front part of the skull, with a sizable metal fragment lying just above the right eye. From this head wound two small irregularly shaped fragments of metal were recovered and turned over to the FBI.

The autopsy also disclosed a wound near the base of the back of President Kennedy's neck slightly to the right of his spine. The doctors traced the course of the bullet through the body* and, as information was received from Parkland Hospital, concluded that the bullet had emerged from the front portion of the President's neck that had been cut away by the tracheotomy at Parkland. The nature and characteristics of this neck wound and the two head wounds are discussed fully in the next chapter.

After the autopsy was concluded at approximately 11 p.m., the President's body was prepared for burial. This was finished at approximately 4 a.m. Shortly thereafter, the President's wife, family and aides left Bethesda Naval Hospital. The President's body was taken to the East Room of the White House where it was placed under ceremonial military guard.

An Early Critique of the Postmortem Examination

In 1966, Doctor Cyril Wecht, coroner of Allegheny County, Pennsylvania, published a cogent critique of the investigation into the assassination of John F. Kennedy (Curran and Shapiro, 1970, pp. 202-216). The cause and manner of death of the President are clear: cause of death, gunshot wound in the head;

---

*This statement is simply not true. The pathologists were ordered by an unknown general, not a medical officer, to refrain from any dissection of the neck and thus a tracing of the bullet course from the upper back wound to wherever it went. (C.G.W.)

manner, homicide. Supporting details however are missing or vague; among these are included range, number of bullets fired, entrance and exit wounds, direction of the bullets, and angle of the bullet paths.

The only biomedical facts available to scholarly critics of the investigation are to be found in the Report and Hearings of the investigating Commission and in the records at Parkland Memorial Hospital of the medical and surgical treatment given to Kennedy and to Connally. There is persuasive evidence that the pathological findings, uncovered by armed forces physicians assigned to do the autopsy, have been edited, modified, and even subjected to deletions before publication was permitted.

The first question to ask is whether the autopsy performed on President Kennedy was complete. Wecht (Curran and Shapiro, 1970) said "By standards found in most competent medical-legal investigative facilities, the autopsy report would not be deemed to be a complete one." The end result has been numerous questions of critical importance to the case not being answered. Some of the questions follow.

The blood type of the President apparently was not known or certainly not given to the Parkland Memorial Hospital doctors who were treating him; he was thus transfused with type 0 Rh negative blood. His wounds were so serious that the blood transfusion was virtually meaningless. Why was the blood type of the President not a matter of ready record on his person, by his personal physician, and by Secret Service personnel accompanying him.?

The emergency treatment given the stricken President at Parkland Memorial Hospital is beyond reproach. No treatment procedures available then or subsequently developed would have had any useful effect on the outcome of the President's wounding.

When the President was finally pronounced legally dead, there should have been a complete external examination of the entire body to catalogue *all* the wounds visible and to describe them anatomically. The fact that the remains were completely disrobed and wrapped in sheets for transportation, in a casket, away from the hospital makes the oversight perplexing. The autopsy report includes no mention of the clothing on the body nor are sketches or photos of the President's clothing included in the final autopsy report despite military directives that such should be done.

Wecht is of the opinion that there was nothing wrong in spiriting the body feloniously out of the legal jurisdiction of the coroner in Dallas in violation of Texas law. His arguments are not convincing. There is every reason to contend that had the Secret Service and other federal officials not flouted Texas law by deceit and threats of violence, a proper postmortem examination would have been made and in all probability the deluge of unbelief would have been prevented.

The autopsy itself performed at Bethesda Naval Hospital was doomed to be defective for a number of reasons.

1. Military doctors alone, subject to orders of superiors, performed the autopsy and allegedly wrote the final draft of the protocol.

2. The autopsy doctors did not consult with the emergency room doctors at Parkland Memorial Hospital *before* they began their examination of the remains.

3. All the clinical information available on the case was not reviewed by the pathologists *before* the anatomical procedures were begun.

4. The clothing worn by the President when the shooting occurred was apparently not available for examination by the pathologists until months after the autopsy was completed and the final report filed.

5. The two Navy pathologists assigned to the autopsy were competent general hospital pathologists, but not competent as forensic pathologists. Lt. Col. Pierre Finck, MC, U.S. Army, was a trained and certified forensic pathologist.

6. At the time of the autopsy some of the world's leading forensic pathologists and gunshot wound experts were located within sixty minutes flight time of the nation's capital: Russell Fisher, M.D., Baltimore; Joseph Spelman, M.D., Philadelphia; Milton Helpern, M.D., New York City; Goeffrey Mann, M.D., Richmond; Alan Moritz,

M.D., Cleveland. None were called in even as an observer of the autopsy; oddly enough a strange assortment of non-medical personnel were apparently permitted in the work room quite contrary to military directives and good autopsy practice.

7. Admiral Burkley autocratically decided to edit the draft of the autopsy report and to release only those portions of it that he deemed "necessary." His incompetence to know what is "necessary and important in a forensic autopsy is demonstrated by the fact that he edited out material information.

8. Contrary to military directives, autopsy photographs and x-rays were not included as integral parts of the final protocol. They were never made available to the autopsy pathologists in preparation of the report or of their testimony before the Commission lawyers.

SOME DIFFICULTIES

Paulette Cooper (1973) has summarized some of the problems associated with the official investigation of the John F. Kennedy assassination.

Three military officers commissioned in the service as doctors were called upon to perform the autopsy on the late President. These physicians, who were military officers, included Commander James J. Humes of the United States Navy Medical Service, Commander J. Thornton Boswell also of the Navy Medical Service, and Lt. Col. Pierre Finck who was an Army officer in the Army Medical Service. None of these physicians had practical firsthand experience of any extent with bullet wounds. The Navy doctors were hospital pathologists. They were qualified to carry out autopsy examinations on patients who had died in military hospitals. The available evidence indicates that these two Navy doctors had only one case of a gunshot wound to their credit before being asked to perform the autopsy on the late President John F. Kennedy. Doctor Pierre Finck was what might be called an administrative pathologist. He reviewed cases of gunshot wounds that were filed by other physicians in the records of the Armed Forces Institute of Pathology. He published in scientific journals material which he was able to extract from the files of the Armed Forces Institute of Pathology. According to the record available, his experience with gunshot wound *at the autopsy table* was limited. Thus one might anticipate from the very beginning of this investigation difficulty, confusion, and inadequate medicolegal investigation.

Such difficulties, in fact arose. The highly skilled surgeons in Parkland Memorial Hospital, Dallas, Texas, first saw the wound in the President's throat just below the larynx (the voice box or the Adam's apple in popular terminology). They described this wound in the anterior neck of the President as being about 3 to 5 millimeters in diameter or about 0.2 of an inch in diameter. Such a hole is rather small. It is compatible with the entrance hole of a bullet. Indeed, several of the surgeons at Parkland Memorial Hospital referred to the wound in the anterior neck of the President as an entrance wound of a bullet.

The doctors who performed the autopsy described a wound in the President's back as being from 4 to 5 millimeters in diameter. This wound was obviously larger than the one in the anterior part of the neck. It is a proper question to ask why the alleged entrance wound in the President's body was larger than the exit wound. Such a situation may occur; it is usually seen in contact wounds of the skull where the skin is stretched tightly over a base of bone. It is uncommon in distant wounds made through soft tissue.

Doctor Cyril Wecht has suggested that there is a good reason to conclude that the late President's wound in the anterior part of the neck is really an entrance wound, as several of the attending surgeons for the moribund President maintained. Doctor Wecht further suggests that the wound in the President's back, which he was able to examine only in photographs, seems to have characteristics of a gunshot wound.

There is further confusion connected with the location of the wound in the President's back. Its position was changed in different versions of the autopsy report and in the official report published by the Commission. The chart done at the scene of the autopsy shows the wound in the back to be located about

4 to 6 inches below the neck. In one version of the autopsy report itself, the pathologists maintain that the wound is at the nape of the neck. On the other hand, the holes in the President's suit coat and in his shirt indicate clearly that these holes are about 6 inches below the top of the collar.

Where, then, was the hole in the President's back? It has been suggested that the President was waving his arms to the crowd and that this motion hiked up his jacket and shirt so that the holes were lined up with a real hole in the skin at the nape of his neck.

Photographs allegedly made at the time the shot occurred indicate that the President did not have his hands up in the air waving to the crowd; rather he was sitting in a relaxed position with his arms on the armrest of the automobile. Even if he were waving his arms to the crowd, the shirt would not have been hiked up as some individuals suggest. The suit coat might very well have been, but then one would anticipate different distances measured on the ruffled up suit coat and the smooth underlying shirt. These differences do not exist.

Moreover, it is difficult to understand how a bullet which entered 4 inches below the neck in the back could exit slightly below the larnyx or Adam's apple in the front of the throat and still originate at a point behind and *above* the President's head. The two wounds described as entrance and exit wounds in the President's body would have required an upward course of the bullet through the President's body. The suggestion has been made that the bullet hit something in the body and ricocheted upward. However, the Warren Commission emphasized several times that the bullet that they claim entered the President's back and came out his throat struck no bone, but in effect slid between masses of muscle. X-rays made of the President's body were reported to show no broken bones in the trunk of the body.

One cannot argue that the President was leaning forward so that the track of the bullet could be explained by the President's position at the time the nonfatal shot struck him. At the time of the shooting, the President could not lean forward because he was wearing a canvas brace which had metal stays in it. This brace was wrapped with an Ace bandage. In this rigid frame he had to sit upright. This device was necessary because of the severe back disability suffered by the late President Kennedy.

Of greater difficulty is the single bullet theory proposed by the Warren Commission. This theory maintains that the bullet that is said to have entered the President's back and gone out through the front of his throat then made a right-angle turn in midair; it went into the Governor's body in the extreme right part of his chest tearing out a portion of his fifth rib. From there it went downward, smashing his right wrist which happened to be resting on his left thigh, and entered his thigh, leaving a chunk of metal in the thigh bone. That same bullet was said to have fallen out of the wound in his left thigh.

It is true that bullets do strange and unexpected things and describe weird patterns in body tissues. But in the air this kind of erratic behavior by bullets is not observed. In the air bullets follow the normal laws of physics that govern all flying objects.

Governor Connally himself had time to turn around when he heard the first shot and maintained, as did his wife who was sitting next to him in the presidential limousine, that it was "inconceivable" that he was struck with the same bullet that hit Kennedy.

The bullet which is said to have done all this damage to two individuals probably weighed somewhere between 160 and 161 grains before it was fired. After allegedly going through seven layers of skin plus two large bones, it weighed 159 grains. Moreover, this bullet was said to have been discovered in a virtually undeformed condition. The bullet said to have performed this pattern was found under strange circumstances on a stretcher in Parkland Memorial Hospital some time after the actual shooting. It showed the engraving of rifling marks on its side. Its nose was undeformed and there was no indication whatever that it had struck bone. Moreover, there was no indication in the written record of the Report or of the Hearings that any tissue or blood was recovered and analyzed from this bullet. Thus it is that if the one bullet theory proposed by the Warren Commission is true, a most remarkable situation obtained. Most bullets, when they strike bone, are deformed; in the process the deformed bullets lose significant amounts of metal as they pass through the bone. Metal particles were reported in the x-rays taken of Governor Connally's wrist and thigh; there were alleged to be metal particles left in the President's body. If the undeformed pristine bullet had lost such a small amount of weight as the Warren Commission reported, it was not in keeping with the laws of physics that it could have caused all the harm it was said to have caused.

On page 60 of the Report of the President's Commission on the Assassination of President Kennedy it was said, "The autopsy also disclosed a wound near the base of the back of President Kennedy's neck slightly to the right of his spine. The doctors traced the course of the bullet through the body and, as information was received from Parkland Hospital, concluded that the bullet had emerged from the front portion of the President's neck that had been cut away by the tracheotomy at Parkland."

The facts as presented in the testimony of the pathologists and government agents who were observers at the autopsy did not support the claim that the pathologists traced the path of the bullet through the body. Quite to the contrary, Doctor Finck, the Army pathologist, stated that he could find no path for the bullet entering the back; he reached a cul-de-sac after a few inches when he probed the wound with his finger. Later, at another legal function, he testified under oath that he and his pathologists had been ordered *not* to dissect the wound in the back-throat region. Without such dissection and without any probing reported, it is not apparent how the path of the bullet could have been traced.

A further misstatement is found in the excerpt quoted from page 60 of the Report, the suggestion that the throat wound was "cut away" in order to insert a tracheotomy tube. Available information indicates that the punctate wound in the throat was "extended" in order to admit the tube. If indeed the wound were "cut away," who did it? Why? When? Where? Medical records from Parkland Memorial Hospital gave no support to the cutting away of the throat wound.

There is a peculiar aspect of the throat wound in the President. It is clear enough that it was, as originally seen, a small punctate hole with no rough or torn edges. Because of a justifiable response to an emergency, the attending surgeons enlarged the wound by cutting through the edges so that a breathing tube could be inserted into the President's trachea.

Because of this operation the autopsy pathologists allegedly could not interpret the throat wound with any degree of certainty. The details of *why not* were never revealed. Had actual tissue been sliced away in the process of inserting the tube or in removing it after the President's death? Was any attempt made to approximate the cut edges so as to reconstruct as much as possible the original punctate hole? If not, why not, since reportedly at that stage the body was not embalmed? Were microscope sections made from the edges of the original hole to ascertain the configuration of the tissues there? Such sections can be stained with many reagents to reveal the presence of foreign material. Such slides can be subjected to x-ray examination, which would reveal metal particles in the wound tract — a device recommended by the Armed Forces Institute of Pathology for certain types of gunshot wounds.

Nowhere in the Report or the Hearings volumes was any indication given that the pathologists attempted to approximate the cut edges of the extended throat wound in order to ascertain whether the original entrancelike bullet hole could be reconstructed. Such a procedure should be routine in a case of this sort. Careful pulling together of the skin flaps with due recognition of how the Langer's lines of cleavage run in that immediate area might well have revealed the probable configuration of the extended wound before it was modified. Photographs of the reconstruction should have been a routine part of the autopsy record.

An even more disastrous oversight on the part of the pathologists was the failure to consult with the doctors at Parkland Hospital *before* any aspect of the autopsy was begun. Such consultation is customary (and indeed is so directed in the official military *Autopsy Manual*) for the chief pathologist at a medicolegal autopsy to obtain as complete a clinical and crime scene digest as is possible, on a firsthand basis, before proceeding with the actual scientific investigation of the corpse.

This obvious consultation did not take place. The results of that neglect are now part of the inadequate and misleading Report of the Commission.

Some mitigation of the questionable autopsy findings might have been obtained had the attending doctors, in consultation with the pathologists and without the hostile presence of any of the Commission staff (calling in outside experts as needed, e.g. Doctor Milton Helpern of New York City or Doctor LeMoyne Schneider of Cincinnati), gone over the autopsy protocol in draft, compared it with the treatment records in the emergency room at Parkland Hospital, and then come up with an orderly and reliable medicolegal report as a scientific body. Needless to say, *all* the photographs and x-rays and rough drafts of notes and sketches would have been part of the data to go over.

The burning of notes and drafts of the autopsy by one or more of the pathologists is astonishing and completely out of keeping with elementary scientific behavior.

Do these comments throw into question the integrity of the pathologists? Do the oversights and unprofessional operations imply fraud or deceit on the part of the pathologists? The answer must be no. Most of the trouble stems from the lack of experience of the pathologists in the specialty of gunshot wounds, especially in the civilian milieu. Two Navy hospital pathologists and an Army research pathologist (all qualified in anatomical pathology) were asked to do a demanding and highly technical postmortem examination in an explosively important case under confused and tense conditions over which they had no control. It is a wonder that the autopsy report is as good as it is.

It is important to recognize clearly that the entire atmosphere created at the Bethesda Naval Hospital the night of the autopsy was one of secrecy and "security." It is also clear that those in charge were not going to permit the "whole truth" to come out. In this peculiar situation one must include the highest ranks of the Department of Defense, notably the Navy, the Secret Service, the FBI, and mysterious generals in and out of uniform whose names are now forgotten but who seemed to have been giving orders that night.

A matter of the gravest importance in the evaluation of the medicolegal investigation of John F. Kennedy's murder is the strange, unscientific, and rightly suspicious manner in which primary data were handled. The hiding away of the x-rays of the autopsy after they were seen briefly that night by the pathologists is a positive action that can be explained only as planned suppression of evidence with obvious aims of deception.

Numerous black and white photographs as well as color photographs were exposed the night of the autopsy and then spirited away by presumed Secret Service agents and hidden somewhere. A roll of film exposed by a Navy enlisted technician was destroyed by some government "agent." To compound what looks like a felony of mass proportions was the Commission's denial to the pathologists of any access to the photographic and x-ray evidence in the preparation of the critical medicolegal testimony. There can be no excuse for this kind of malicious manipulation of events. The Commission and its staff knew individually and as a body that the photographs and x-rays were essential to a meaningful description of the autopsy and its interpretation. Doctor Humes on the stand clearly told the Commission that the sketches (made by a Navy enlisted man who had never seen the body nor the photographs nor the x-rays) could not be accurate and that he could not testify to any useful details without the photographs.

Again the pathologists cannot be faulted in this deception. They were caught in a maelstrom created by ruthless men who had the power and lack of morals that permitted them to manipulate history.

In the process of suppression of evidence, those responsible effectively erased the possibility of ever getting precise information on the most tragic event of this century. The validity of the photographs as evidence of anything was so compromised by secrecy, apparent wanderings from government to private files and back, and loss by government agencies that even their historical value has been diminished. The greatest crime was that the Commission aided and abetted this monstrous deception by not bringing into the light of day *all* the primary evidence and insuring its validity when such was possible. Minutes of secret meetings of the Commission revealed that they knew the evidential value of the photographs but refused to include them in the record. Most of the junk in the twenty-six volumes of Exhibits and Hearings could be thrown out with no loss if only the basic data provided by x-rays and photographs taken at the autopsy table were included with minute evaluations provided by the pathologists.

In an attempt to justify the suppression and possible destruction of primary and critical evidence, appeals have been made by Commission members to "good taste," "sensitivities," and other inane reasons (Warren himself so appealed). Defenders of the Commission Report use similar excuses. Such attempts to justify suppression of basic scientific data in a murder investigation are silly, stupid, or further evidence of maliciousness.

In the summary Report of the Presidential Commission on the Assassination of President Kennedy (p. 54), it was stated that "When Dr. Perry noted free air and blood in the President's chest cavity, he asked that chest tubes be inserted to allow for drainage of blood and air. Drs. Paul C. Peters and Charles R. Baxter initiated these procedures." Specifically, chest drainage tubes were inserted into the dying President's body. This work was done, under the direction of the highly skilled surgeon Doctor Perry, by two other doctors who were also, according to the information available, skilled surgeons.

Therefore, the lack of any penetration by bullet or by surgical instruments into the chest cavity, according to the autopsy pathologist, is confusing. What do the photographs of the internal wall of the late President's chest cavity reveal?

A preliminary conference between the autopsy pathologists and the surgeons at Parkland Memorial Hospital who treated the stricken President would have helped to obviate some of the confusion about postmortem findings. Such conference is a normal and standard procedure in any criminal case.

The Clothing

A source of confusion is the testimony of Doctor Humes that

the hole in the back of the President's suit coat was about 6 inches below the top of the collar and about 2 inches to the right of the center seam of the coat. According to page 92 of the summary Report, an FBI agent, Frazier, observed a "roughly" circular hole about 1/4 inch in diameter, located in the rear of the coat, 5 3/8 inches below the top of the collar, and 1 3/4 inches to the right of the center seam along the back of the coat. The Report admitted that the precise size of the bullet could not be determined from that hole, but claims that it was consistent with having been made by a 6.5 millimeter bullet. That statement, of course, is meaningless because the hole could be consistent with a number of different calibers having made it.

In the summary Report, it was also stated (p. 92) "The shirt worn by the President contained a hole on the backside five and three-quarter inches below the top of the collar, and one and one-eighth inch to the right of the middle of the back of the shirt. The hole in the rear of the shirt was approximately circular in shape, and about one-fourth of an inch in diameter with the fibers pressed inward." The conclusion in the summary Report was that this was an entrance hole. It was also assumed that the holes in the suit jacket and in the shirt were made by the same bullet.

A minor problem arose because in the testimony of Doctor Humes, reference was made to the "center seam" along the back of the shirt. In the summary Report, reference was made only to the middle of the back of the shirt. It would be helpful if the exact positioning of the hole in the back of the shirt from right to left were made with reference to a more stable point. If there were no midseam, then the seams of the nearest and farthest sleeve should have been points of reference.

With respect to the hole in the front of the shirt, the summary Report said the following. "On the front of the shirt, examination revealed a hole seven-eighths of an inch below the collar button and a similar opening seven-eighths of an inch below the buttonhole. These two holes fell into alinement on overlapping positions when the shirt was buttoned. Each hole was a vertical, ragged slit approximately one-half of an inch in height with the cloth fibers protruding outward. Although the characteristics of the slit established that the missile had exited to the front, the irregular nature of the slit precluded a positive determination that it was a bullet hole." Were one to place this shirt on a mannequin and line up the hole in the back of the shirt with the holes in the front of the shirt, the angle at which the bullet actually travelled through the President's body would not be very close to the angle that the bullet would have had to travel were the theory of the single bullet proposed by the Commission, in fact, the true explanation of one wound in the President and the wounding of Governor Connally.

Examination of the Brain

Instructions for the examination of the brain as an integral part of a complete autopsy are explicit in the military *Autopsy Manual.* After the skull has been opened properly, the brain is removed. Then "fix the brain and spinal cord in 10 percent formalin." It is the experience of many pathologists that 10 percent *neutral* formalin (pH 7.0 and buffered) should be used. Thus, if samples of the fixed brain are used for microscopic studies there will be no formalin interference with clean staining of the sections. "The brain should be allowed to harden in fixative for at least one week, preferably two weeks, before sectioning. The fixing fluid should be changed during the first 24 hours and at the end of one week."

Provision is made for the requirement of a rapid diagnosis. "If immediate diagnosis is necessary, the brain may be cut in the fresh state. This procedure is expedited if the freshly sectioned surface is pressed firmly against a piece of glass before the next cut is made, and the knife blade is flooded with 95 percent alcohol."

Of special interest to any evaluation of an autopsy performed under military auspices is the statement, "If desired, the intact fixed brain may be forwarded to the Armed Forces Institute of Pathology." That institute is one of the glories of American medicine. It is world-famous for its outstanding work in pathological research, teaching, consultation, and service. It is operated as a triservice medical institute devoted to the teaching and investigation of important matters in pathology. Its benefits to the nation and indeed to mankind generally are incalculable. It is a human resource that at all costs must be preserved, strengthened, and supported.

Had the brain been turned over to the Armed Forces Institute of Pathology for exhaustive study, a competent, incontrovertible report would have resulted and there would have been no disappearing act on the part of the brain as has occurred.

Internal evidence from the autopsy report and from the supplement leads to the conclusion that the brain was not sent to the Armed Forces Institute of Pathology for detailed study. Why not? Certainly the evaluation of the brain injury to the late President deserved nothing but the most complete and sophisticated probing that could be done, throwing into the study every technical and scientific resource available in this country. In view of the fact that one of the pathologists was a staff member of the Armed Forces Institute of Pathology and one other had taken at least one pathology course there, the total by-passing of that unique resource defies understanding.

The *Autopsy Manual* available to all military medical service personnel goes on to explain how a brain should be properly dissected for adequate study and diagnosis. "When the brain has hardened in fixative it should be cut in coronal sections not more than 1 cm in thickness. Place the brain on a dissecting board with the ventral surface upward so that the landmarks of the base can be used in orienting the coronal cuts symmetrically. Remove the brain stem and cerebellum with a thin knife, cutting across the cerebral peduncles in a plane perpendicular to the axis of the brain stem and aqueduct. Begin the parallel coronal sections of the cerebral hemispheres at the frontal poles. The brain stem and cerebellum together are cut by parallel sections 0.5 cm apart in a plane perpendicular to the axis of the brain stem."

Clearly that sort of professional examination was not done on the murdered President's brain for what certainly seems a frivolous excuse, i.e. in the interest of preserving the specimen.

Restrictions on the Autopsy Record

The written record of the autopsy clearly suggests that the

pathologists involved did a dismal job; the performance was not up to the minimal standards demanded in the *Autopsy Manual,* which is the official directive for physicians in the Departments of the Army, the Navy, and the Air Force. However, one must realize that they were military officers on active duty. The charitable view would be to suggest that they were not allowed to reveal all the facts that they found. It seems to be a safe contention that their report was changed at some date after it was written. It also seems evident that during the actual autopsy they were under some kind of unethical control, probably by the Secret Service Agency or by the military.

This suggestion has merit when one examines the sworn testimony of Doctor Finck (the Army pathologist at Kennedy's autopsy) made at the trial in New Orleans of Clay Shaw. Doctor Finck was asked why the pathologists did not carry out the routine, standard, ordinary task of dissecting the bullet wound in the President's back. This dissection would have revealed the path of the bullet. Doctor Finck testified under oath that the pathologists were told not to dissect the wound. He further swore that this order was given to them by some general whose name he had forgotten. How such a situation could have come about is hard to understand at this time. The fact remains, it did occur.

It is known that the complete autopsy report as written by the pathologists was altered during its route through military channels. Certain sections of the report were removed. Admiral George Burkley, who was President Kennedy's personal physician, admitted that he doctored the autopsy report. What happened to the first report that went to Admiral Burkley? He had it two months before he released portions of the autopsy protocol. Parts of the autopsy report were probably destroyed at some time.

This suggestion is not a frivolous one, because the first report that was written, the apparent original draft that indicated where the bullets went into the body and exited the body, the report that stated where the wounds were, how many bullets there were, and the paths of these bullets, the report that indicated whether or not any bullets were still in Kennedy's body, was burned by Doctor Humes, who admitted writing this original version. Admiral Burkley certified to this most unusual procedure for a pathologist and a scientist to carry out. It is difficult if not impossible to understand how the original draft of such an important autopsy could have been burned. The burning was not accidental. The burning was willful and was so recorded and sworn to.

These actions raise a question about the peculiarity of certain missing facts. For example, it is known that the pathologists actually examined President Kennedy's adrenal glands. Doctor Boswell, one of the pathologists at the autopsy, admitted that the adrenal glands were identified. Were they diseased? One must conclude firmly that they were diseased and probably showed that the late President suffered from severe Addison's disease. If they had not been diseased, the doctors involved and the politicians would have been happy to have discussed these healthy adrenal glands at great length.

Could it be that the large unidentified object seen in the photograph of the President's brain was in fact a tumor (either benign or malignant) that was the root cause of his adrenal problems? Paulette Cooper (1973) concluded her evaluation of the Warren Commission Report with this paragraph. "But these are speculations which may never be satisfied because the parts of the body that could prove or disprove them — the brain — is missing, together with vital portions of the autopsy report. Withholding or altering information has fostered exactly what the public and the government would have preferred ended: rumors, theories, and insinuations of conspiracy."

In a handwritten draft of the autopsy on President Kennedy's remains written by Commander James J. Humes, who was the chief autopsy pathologist, there are several interesting statements (Commission Exhibit No. 397).

The anterior neck wound observed in Parkland Hospital was called a "puncture wound" of the low anterior neck approximately in the midline. "A tracheotomy was performed by extending the latter wound." Further it was reported that "an injury to the rt. lateral wall of the trachea was observed."

"Situated on the upper rt. posterior thorax just above the upper border of the scapula there is a 7 x 14 mm oval (crossed out) wound. This wound is measured to be 14 cm from the tip of the right acromion process and 14 cm below the tip of the rt. mastoid process."

Situated in the low anterior neck at approximately the level of the third and fourth tracheal rings is a 6.5 cm long transverse wound with widely gaping irregular edges." This was the appearance of what once was a round hole after being modified in the process of emergency procedures administered to the dying President. Only the emergency room surgeons could ever testify about the appearance of the throat wound. For the pathologists it no longer existed.

Addison's Disease

It was rumored that President Kennedy had a form of Addison's disease. Clinically the disease is primary adrenal cortical insufficiency. It afflicts about 1 person in every 100,000 of population. It is caused by destruction or atrophy (wasting away) of the adrenal cortex. "Clinical adrenal insufficiency usually does not occur unless at least 90 per cent of the adrenal cortex has been destroyed" (Liddle, 1975).

The disease usually arises accompanied by other pathological conditions. Victims of the disease in the autoimmune form have an unusually high incidence of diabetes mellitus, hypothyroidism, and hypoparathyroidism. The physiological results of Addison's disease are all explainable in terms of deficient amounts of cortisol, aldosterone, and adrenal androgen in the patient's body.

One sign of the disease apparent to the victim as well as to his friends is the characteristic discoloration of the skin. The skin has a dingy or smoky look; it may show a variety of tints of deep amber or chestnut brown. The discoloration has been called a suntan that does not wear off. Adequate medical treatment may forestall the discoloration and even erase that which may have already developed.

Modern medical tests can demonstrate early and precisely the existence of the disease. Treatment with powerful drugs and the liberal intake of table salt in all its forms by the addisonian patient can insure normal activity and life expectancy. Associated diseases, however, may modify the prognosis. Stressful situations are always a threat to the patient with Addison's disease.

Implications of the Death Certificate

The alleged death certificate that was signed by Rear Admiral G.G. Burkley states clearly that a wound was found "in the posterior back at about the level of the third thoracic vertebra" (see Newcomb and Adams, 1974). A senior medical officer in the Navy with years of experience as a physician obviously would know how to describe the anatomical location of a wound, especially when it was located in one of his regular patients. Therefore, it seems probable that the back wound in the late President was at the level of the third thoracic vertebra.

Assuming that the nonfatal bullet entered Kennedy's back as the death certificate stated, where would it go? If one were to line up a point at the level of the third thoracic vertebra on the back with the point where the Warren Commission concluded the bullet exited at the anterior throat region, perhaps the line could be extended in both directions to work out a bullet path from the anatomical data.

According to Doctor Humes' description of the anterior neck wound, it was low in the anterior portion of the neck at the level of the third and forth tracheal rings.

Therefore, two points define the line of the track of the non-fatal bullet that went through Kennedy: a point just to the right of the backbone and at the level of the third thoracic vertebra on the back, and a second point about midline in the throat but at the level of the third cartilage ring below the larynx.

Such a line would have had a direction from front to back with an angle slightly above the horizontal. If the bullet entering the back moved forward in a horizontal direction, it would have struck the manubrium of the sternum (the upper part of the breastbone). If the angle of the bullet entering the back were downward, the bullet could not have come out at the level of the third or fourth tracheal ring. It would have struck the middle of the body of the sternum. If the bullet entered the body at an angle to the right or left but in a slightly downward course, it would have hit the muscles between the first and second ribs and those between the second and third ribs on either the right or left side of the second piece of the sternum.

In order for the nonfatal bullet to tear the trachea as it did and yet enter the back at the level of the third thoracic vertebra, an upward course of the bullet track seems to have been required, especially since the late President was held rigidly upright by a medical body brace.

Either the throat wound and the back wound were not in communication and were separate and distinct wounds, or the angle of the bullet track would have to be reworked to give a more nearly horizontal or even upward course. The Warren Commission in its Report (p. 106) gave an angle of around 17 to 18 degrees downward as the course through the President's body. The relative locations of the back wound and the throat wound do not support that conclusion.

Discrepancies in the autopsy are summarized in Table 5-I.

Table 5-I

COMPARING THE OBSERVATIONS REQUIRED BY
ARMED FORCES AUTOPSY MANUAL
WITH OBSERVATIONS MADE AT J.F. KENNEDY AUTOPSY

Observation	Autopsy Manual	Gross JFK Autopsy
Clinical abstract	detailed	incomplete
Every organ to be examined	yes	no reference
Description of exterior	detailed	no reference
Organs of neck: thyroid,	detailed	no reference
parathyroid, larynx, pharynx	mandatory	no reference
Lungs	yes	cut surface limited to one lobe
Heart	yes	yes
Aorta and vessels	yes	incomplete
Spleen	yes	no reference

Liver	detailed	no reference
Gall bladder and ducts	yes	no reference
Pancreas	detailed	no reference
Adrenals	size, cut surface	no reference
Gastrointestinal tract	detailed	superficial
Genitourinary tract	complete details of all parts	no reference
Seminal vesicles, prostate, testes	yes	no reference
Muscles, bones, joints	yes	single sentence
Head	yes	partial
Brain	detailed	external surface only
Cord	yes	no reference
Temporal bone	yes	no reference
Ear	yes	no reference
Skull sinus	yes	no reference
Eyes	yes	no reference
Bone marrow	yes	no reference
	Microscopic	*Microscopic*
Heart	detailed	very general
Lungs	detailed	very general
Liver	detailed, plus gall bladder	general, no gall bladder
Pancreas	yes	no reference
Spleen	yes	very general
Adrenals	complete	no reference
Kidneys	detailed	general
Pelvic organs	all	none
Lymphatic system	detailed	no reference
Thyroid	complete	no reference
Bone marrow	detailed	no reference
Trabecular bone	yes	no reference
Brain: meninges, parenchyma, vessels, perivascular infiltrations, ependyma	complete	random pieces with vague comments
	Other	*Other*
Photographs*	"Photographs should be made in all medico-legal autopsies. . . ."	not certain; claimed to have been made but apparently poor quality.
Clothing	details of disturbances of all clothing	no

*Autopsy manual (p. 56) directs that "the photographs made by the pathologist should be attached to the final autopsy report."

Observation	Other	Other
Blood group	yes	no reference
Blood for alcohol	yes	no reference
Fingerprints	yes	no reference

Where Was the Back Wound?

If one were to take a human male of the approximate size of the late John F. Kennedy and position the wound in the back as described in words by the Warren Commission, the bullet hole would be located just to the right of the transverse process of the seventh cervical vertebra. The death certificate executed by Admiral Burkley, the late President's personal physician, stated that the bullet hole in the back was located at the level of the third thoracic vertebra, a place in accord with the bullet holes in the back of the suit coat and the shirt. Why the discrepancy with respect to where the hole was?

The discrepancy between the location of the hole in the President's back as concluded by the Commission and the known location of the hole as evidenced by the suit coat and the shirt has been explained as the result of the coat's being hiked up toward the head while the President was presumably waving to the crowd.

Such explanation may account for the suit coat hole being out of line with the "true" hole; the explanation is not workable with the shirt hole. The shirt would not have been hiked up nearly 6 inches as a result of the President's waving. Photographs taken moments before the first shot indicate that the late President's arm was resting on the limousine armrest and was not extended to any great degree.

Some Legal Snarls

According to Texas law, the body of a victim of homicide may not be moved out of the county of his death until an autopsy is completed on the remains. The death certificate is signed by the coroner having jurisdiction. A physician who happened to have rendered first aid or emergency room treatment to a homicide victim is not competent, as a result of his ministrations, to sign the death certificate.

This pattern is a general one in most states. All responsible police officers are familiar with these requirements. It cannot be denied that at least some of the federal police and officials at Dallas in 1963 were clearly aware of the law.

Despite the clear-cut, routine, and unquestionably justified provisions of Texas law in regard to autopsies on homicide victims, John F. Kennedy's remains were spirited away from the legal authority of the Dallas coroner and transported to Bethesda, Maryland where an autopsy was performed.

The role of violence, threats of violence, deceit, and the flouting of the law on the part of federal officials who engineered the transport of Kennedy's remains deserves serious study by scholars.

Witnesses to the Autopsy

No civilian forensic pathologists or forensic science experts were involved at any time in the autopsy as observers, consultants, assistants, or otherwise insofar as official records reveal.

The record does reveal the presence of a number of unidentified persons in the autopsy room. Some were clearly not medical personnel; others may have been. The reasons for their presence were not recorded.

The autopsy report with its supplement was printed in the Report of the Warren Commission. These documents are quoted verbatim in the section immediately following.

CLINICAL SUMMARY:

According to available information the deceased, President John F. Kennedy, was riding in an open car in a motorcade during an official visit to Dallas, Texas on 22 November 1963. The President was sitting in the right rear seat with Mrs. Kennedy seated on the same seat to his left. Sitting directly in front of the President was Governor John B. Connally of Texas and directly in front of Mrs. Kennedy sat Mrs. Connally. The vehicle was moving at a slow rate of speed down an incline into an underpass that leads to a freeway route to

AUTOPSY REPORT (COMMISSION EXHIBIT NUMBER 387)

Standard Form 503
Revised August 1954
Promulgated
By Bureau of the Budget
Circular A—32 (Rev.)

CLINICAL RECORD	AUTOPSY PROTOCOL	A63-272 (JJH:ec)		

Date and Hour Died	A.M. P.M.	Date and Hour Autopsy Performed	A.M. P.M.	CHECK ONE		
22 November 1963 1300(CST)		22 November 1963 2000(EST)		Full Autopsy	Head Only	Trunk Only

Prosector (497831) CDR J. J. HUMES, MC, USN	Assistant (489878) CDR "J" THORNTON BOSWELL, MC,USN	X		

CLINICAL DIAGNOSES *(Including operations)*

LCOL PIERRE A. FINCK, MS, USA (04 043 332)

Ht. - 72 1/2 inches
Wt. - 170 pounds
Eyes - Blue
Hair - Reddish brown

PATHOLOGICAL DIAGNOSES

CAUSE OF DEATH: Gunshot wound, head.

APPROVED-SIGNATURE

J. J. HUMES, CDR, MC, USN

MILITARY ORGANIZATION *(When required)* PRESIDENT, United States	Age 46	Sex Male	Race Cauc.	Identification No.	Autopsy No. A63-272
PATIENT'S IDENTIFICATION *(For typed or written entires give: Name-last, first, middle; grade, date; hospital or medical facility)*		Register No.		Ward No.	

KENNEDY, JOHN F.
NAVAL MEDICAL SCHOOL

AUTOPSY PROTOCOL
Standard Form 503

the Dallas Trade Mart where the President was to deliver an address.

Three shots were heard and the President fell forward bleeding from the head. (Governor Connally was seriously wounded by the same gunfire.) According to newspaper reports ("Washington Post" November 23, 1963) Bob Jackson, a Dallas "Times Herald" Photographer, said he looked around as he heard the shots and saw a rifle barrel disappearing into a window on an upper floor of the nearby Texas School Book Depository Building.

Shortly following the wounding of the two men the car was driven to Parkland Hospital in Dallas. In the emergency room of that hospital the President was attended by Dr. Malcolm Perry. Telephone communication with Dr. Perry on November 23, 1963 develops the following information relative to the observations made by Dr. Perry and procedures performed there prior to death.

Dr. Perry noted the massive wound of the head and a second much smaller wound of the low anterior neck in approximately the midline. A tracheotomy was performed by extending the latter wound. At this point bloody air was noted bubbling from the wound and an injury to the right lateral wall of the trachea was observed. Incisions were made in the upper anterior chest wall bilaterally to combat possible subcutaneous emphysema. Intravenous infusions of blood and saline were begun and oxygen was administered. Despite these measures cardiac arrest occurred and closed chest cardiac massage failed to reestablish cardiac action. The President was pronounced dead approximately thirty to forty minutes after receiving his wounds.

The remains were transported via the Presidential plane to Washington, D. C. and subsequently to the Naval Medical School, National Naval Medical Center, Bethesda, Maryland for postmortem examination.

GENERAL DESCRIPTION OF BODY:

The body is that of a muscular, well-developed and well nourished adult Caucasian male measuring 72 1/2 inches and weighing approximately 170 pounds. There is beginning rigor mortis, minimal dependent livor mortis of the dorsum, and early algor mortis. The hair is reddish brown and abundant, the eyes are blue, the right pupil measuring 8 mm. in diameter, the left 4 mm. There is edema and ecchymosis of the inner canthus region of the left eyelid measuring approximately 1.5 cm. in greatest diameter. There is edema and ecchymosis diffusely over the right supra-orbital ridge with abnormal mobility of the underlying bone. (The remainder of the scalp will be described with the skull.) There is clotted blood on the external ears but otherwise the ears, nares, and mouth are essentially unremarkable. The teeth are in excellent repair and there is some pallor of the oral mucous membrane.

Situated on the upper right posterior thorax just above the upper border of the scapula there is a 7 x 4 millimeter oval wound. This wound is measured to be 14 cm. from the tip of the right acromion process and 14 cm. below the tip of the right mastoid process.

Situated in the low anterior neck at approximately the level fo the third and fourth tracheal rings is a 6.5 cm. long transverse wound with widely gaping irregular edges. (The depth and character of these wounds will be further described below.)

Situated on the anterior chest wall in the nipple line are bilateral 2 cm. long recent transverse surgical incisions into the subcutaneous tissue. The one on the left is situated 11 cm. cephalad to the nipple and the one on the right 8 cm. cephalad to the nipple. There is no hemorrhage or ecchymosis associated with these wounds. A similar clean wound measuring 2 cm. in length is situated on the antero-lateral aspect of the left mid arm. Situated on the antero-lateral aspect of each ankle is a recent 2 cm. transverse incision into the subcutaneous tissue.

There is an old well healed 8 cm. McBurney abdominal incision. Over the lumbar spine in the midline is an old, well healed 15 cm. scar. Situated on the upper antero-lateral aspect of the right thigh is an old, well healed 8 cm. scar.

MISSILE WOUNDS:

1. There is a large irregular defect of the scalp and skull on the right involving chiefly the parietal bone but extending somewhat into the temporal and occipital regions. In this region there is an actual absence of scalp and bone producing a defect which measures approximately 13 cm. in greatest diameter.

From the irregular margins of the above scalp defect tears extend in stellate fashion into the more or less intact scalp as follows:

a. From the right inferior temporo-parietal margin anterior to the right ear to a point slightly above the tragus.

b. From the anterior parietal margin anteriorly on the forehead to approximately 4 cm. above the right orbital ridge.

c. From the left margin of the main defect across the midline antero-laterally for a distance of approximately 8 cm.

d. From the same starting point as c. 10 cm. posterolaterally.

Situated in the posterior scalp approximately 2.5 cm. laterally to the right and slightly above the external occipital protuberance is a lacerated wound measuring 15 x 6 mm. In the underlying bone is a corresponding wound through the skull which exhibits beveling of the margins of the bone when viewed from the inner aspect of the skull.

Clearly visible in the above described large skull defect and exuding from it is lacerated brain tissue which on close inspection proves to represent the major portion of the right cerebral hemisphere. At this point it is noted that the falx cerebri is extensively lacerated with disruption of the superior saggital sinus.

Upon reflecting the scalp multiple complete fracture lines are seen to radiate from both the large defect at the vertex and the smaller wound at the occiput. These vary greatly in length and direction, the longest measuring approximately 19 cm. These result in the production of numerous fragments which vary in size from a few millimeters to 10 cm. in greatest diameter.

The complexity of these fractures and the fragments thus produced tax satisfactory verbal description and are better appreciated in photographs and roentgenograms which are prepared.

The brain is removed and preserved for further study following formalin fixation.

Received as separate specimens from Dallas, Texas are three fragments of skull bone which in aggregate roughly approximate the dimensions of the large defect described above. At one angle of the largest of these fragments is a portion of the perimeter of a roughly circular wound presumably of exit which exhibits beveling of the outer aspect of the bone and is estimated to measure approximately 2.5 to 3.0 cm. in diameter. Roentgenograms of this fragment reveal minute particles of metal in the bone at this margin. Roentgenograms of the skull reveal multiple minute metallic fragments along a line corresponding with a line joining the above described small occipital wound and the right supra-orbital ridge. From the surface of the disrupted right cerebral cortex two small irregularly shaped fragments of metal are recovered. These measure 7 x 2 mm. and 3 x 1 mm. These are placed in the custody of Agents Francis X. O'Neill, Jr. and James W. Sibert, of the Federal Bureau of Investigation, who executed a receipt therefor (attached).

2. The second wound presumably of entry is that described above in the upper right posterior thorax. Beneath the skin there is ecchymosis of subcutaneous tissue and musculature. The missile path through the fascia and musculature cannot be easily probed. The wound presumably of exit was that described by Dr. Malcolm Perry of Dallas in the low anterior cervical region. When observed by Dr. Perry the wound measured "a few millimeters in diameter," however it was extended as a tracheotomy incision and thus its character is distorted at the time of autopsy. However, there is considerable ecchymosis of the strap muscles of the right side of the neck and of the fascia about the trachea adjacent to the line of the tracheotomy wound. The third point of reference in connecting these two wounds is in the apex (supra-clavicular portion) of the right pleural cavity. In this region there is contusion of the parietal pleura and of the extreme apical portion of the right upper lobe of the lung. In both instances the diameter of contusion and ecchymosis at the point of maximal involvement measured 5 cm. Both the visceral and parietal pleura are intact overlying these areas of trauma.

INCISIONS:

The scalp wounds are extended in the coronal plane to examine the cranial content and the customary (**Y**) shaped incision is used to examine the body cavities.

THORACIC CAVITY:

The body cage is unremarkable. The thoracic organs are in their normal positions and relationships and there is no increase in free pleural fluid. The above described area of contusion in the apical portion of the right pleural cavity is noted.

LUNGS:

The lungs are of essentially similar appearance the right weighing 320 Gm., the left 290 Gm. The lungs are well aerated with smooth glistening pleural surfaces and gray-pink color. A 5 cm. diameter area of purplish red discoloration and increased firmness to palpation is situated in the apical portion of the right upper lobe. This corresponds to the similar area described in the overlying parietal pleura. Incision in this region reveals recent hemorrhage into pulmonary parenchyma.

HEART:

The pericardial cavity is smooth walled and contains approximately 10 cc. of straw-colored fluid. The heart is of essentially normal external contour and weighs 350 Gm. The pulmonary artery is opened in situ and no abnormalities are noted. The cardiac chambers contain moderate amounts of postmortem clotted blood. There are no gross abnormalities of the leaflets of any of the cardiac valves. The following are the circumferences of the cardiac valves: aortic 7.5 cm., pulmonic 7 cm., tricuspid 12 cm. mitral 11 cm. The myocardium is firm and reddish brown. The left ventricular myocardium averages 1.2 cm. in thickness, the right ventricular myocardium 0.4 cm. The coronary arteries are dissected and are of normal distribution and smooth walled and elastic throughout.

ABDOMINAL CAVITY:

The abdominal organs are in their normal positions and

relationships and there is no increase in free peritoneal fluid. The vermiform appendix is surgically absent and there are a few adhesions joining the region of the cecum to the ventral abdominal wall at the above described old abdominal incisional scar.

SKELETAL SYSTEM:

Aside from the above described skull wounds there are no significant gross skeletal abnormalities.

PHOTOGRAPH:

Black and white and color photographs depicting significant findings are exposed but not developed. These photographs were placed in the custody of Agent Roy H. Kellerman of the U. S. Secret Service, who executed a receipt therefor (attached).

ROENTGENOGRAMS:

Roentgenograms are made of the entire body and of the separately submitted three fragments of skull bone. These are developed and were placed in the custody of Agent Roy H. Kellerman of the U. S. Secret Service, who executed a receipt therefor (attached).

SUMMARY:

Based on the above observations it is our opinion that the deceased died as a result of two perforating gunshot wounds inflicted by high velocity projectiles fired by a person or persons unknown. The projectiles were fired from a point behind and somewhat above the level of the deceased. The observations and available information do not permit a satisfactory estimate as to the sequence of the two wounds.

The fatal missile entered the skull above and to the right of the external occipital protuberance. A portion of the projectile traversed the cranial cavity in a posterior-anterior direction (see lateral skull roentgenograms) depositing minute particles along its path. A portion of the projectile made its exit through the parietal bone on the right carrying with it portions of cerebrum, skull and scalp. The two wounds of the skull combined with the force of the missile produced extensive fragmentation of the skull, laceration of the superior saggital sinus, and of the right cerebral hemisphere.

The other missile entered the right superior posterior thorax above the scapula and traversed the soft tissues of the supra-scapular and the supra-clavicular portions of the base of the right side of the neck. This missile produced contusions of the right apical parietal pleura and of the apical portion of the right upper lobe of the lung. The missile contused the strap muscles of the right side of the neck, damaged the trachea and made its exit through the anterior surface of the neck. As far as can be ascertained this missile struck no bony structures in its path through the body.

In addition, it is our opinion that the wound of the skull produced such extensive damage to the brain as to preclude the possibility of the deceased surviving the injury.

A supplementary report will be submitted following more detailed examination of the brain and of microscopic sections. However, it is not anticipated that these examinations will materially alter the findings.

/s/	/s/	/s/
J. J. HUMES	"J" THORNTON BOSWELL	PIERRE A. FINCK
CDR, MC, USN (497831)	CDR, MC, USN (489878)	LT COL, MC, USA
		(04-043-322)

At a later date the following supplementary report was filed and became part of the official record.

COMMISSION EXHIBIT NUMBER 391

Supplementary Report of Autopsy Number A63-272
President John F. Kennedy

PATHOLOGICAL EXAMINATION REPORT A63-272

GROSS DESCRIPTION OF BRAIN:

Following formalin fixation the brain weighs 1500 gms.

The right cerebral hemisphere is found to be markedly disrupted. There is a longitudinal laceration of the right hemisphere which is para-sagittal in position approximately 2.5 cm. to the right of the midline which extends from the tip of the occipital lobe posteriorly to the tip of the frontal lobe anteriorly. The base of the laceration is situated approximately 4.5 cm. below the vertex in the white matter. There is considerable loss of cortical substance above the base of the laceration, particularly in the parietal lobe. The margins of this laceration are at all points jagged and irregular, with additional lacerations extending in varying directions and for varying distances from the main laceration. In addition, there is a laceration of the corpus callosum extending from the genu to the tail. Exposed in this latter laceration are the interiors of the right lateral and third ventricles.

When viewed from the vertex the left cerebral hemisphere is intact. There is marked engorgement of meningeal blood vessels of the left temporal and frontal regions with considerable associated sub-arachnoid hemorrhage. The gyri and sulci over the left hemisphere are of essentially normal size and distribution. Those on the right are too fragmented and distorted for satisfactory description.

When viewed from the basilar aspect the disruption of the right cortex is again obvious. There is a longitudinal laceration of the mid-brain through the floor of the third ventricle just behind the optic chiasm and the mammillary bodies. This laceration partially communicates with an oblique 1.5 cm. tear through the left cerebral peduncle. There are irregular superficial lacerations over the basilar aspects of the left temporal and frontal lobes.

In the interest of preserving the specimen coronal sections were not made.* The following sections are taken for microscopic examination:

    a. From the margin of the laceration in the right parietal lobe.

    b. From the margin of the laceration in the corpus callosum.

    c. From the anterior portion of the laceration in the right frontal lobe.

---

*This is a frivolous excuse for not carrying out a routine procedure. The only value of the preserved brain was to give information.

d. From the contused left fronto-parietal cortex.
e. From the line of transection of the spinal cord.
f. From the right cerebellar cortex.
g. From the superficial laceration of the basilar aspect of the left temporal lobe.

During the course of this examination seven (7) black and white and six (6) color 4x5 inch negatives are exposed but not developed (the cassettes containing these negatives have been delivered by hand to Rear Admiral George W. Burkley, [*sic*] MC, USN, White House Physician).

MICROSCOPIC EXAMINATION:
BRAIN:

Multiple sections from representative areas as noted above are examined. All sections are essentially similar and show extensive disruption of the brain tissue with associated hemorrhage. In none of the sections examined are there significant abnormalities other than those directly related to the recent trauma.

HEART:

Sections show a moderate amount of sub-epicardial fat. The coronary arteries, myocardial fibers, and endocardium are unremarkable.

LUNGS:

Sections through the grossly described area of contusion in the right upper lobe exhibit disruption of alveolar walls and recent hemorrhage into alveoli. Sections are otherwise essentially unremarkable.

LIVER:

Sections show the normal hepatic architecture to be well preserved. The parenchymal cells exhibit markedly granular cytoplasm indicating high glycogen content which is characteristic of the "liver biopsy pattern" of sudden death.

SPLEEN:

Sections show no significant abnormalities.

KIDNEYS:

Sections show no significant abnormalities aside from dilatation and engorgement of blood vessels of all calibers.

SKIN WOUNDS:

Sections through the wounds in the occipital and upper right posterior thoracic regions are essentially similar. In each there is loss of continuity of the epidermis with coagulation necrosis of the tissues at the wound margins. The scalp wound exhibits several small fragments of bone at its margins in the sub-cutaneous tissue.

FINAL SUMMARY:

This supplementary report covers in more detail the extensive degree of cerebral trauma in this case. However neither this portion of the examination nor the microscopic examinations alter the previously submitted report or add significant details to the cause of death.

/s/

J. J. Humes
CDR, MC, USN, 497831

6 December 1963

From: Commanding Officer, U. S. Naval Medical School
To: The White House Physician
Via: Commanding Officer, National Naval Medical Center
Subj: Supplementary report of Naval Medical School autopsy No. A63-272, John F. Kennedy; forwarding of
1. All copies of the above subject final supplementary report are forwarded herewith.

/s/

J. H. STROVER, JR.

----

6 December 1963

FIRST ENDORSEMENT
From: Commanding Officer, National Naval Medical Center
To: The White House Physician
1. Forwarded.

C. B. GALLOWAY

Drafts of the Report

A handwritten draft of the autopsy report (by Commander Humes) was printed in the Hearings and Exhibits of the Commission. Precisely what draft it was cannot be certain.

The record is clear that extensive editing, which included deletions, took place before the final draft was published. The reasons for these editorial changes are not clear. The excuses made for the fact of editing are frivolous and hardly forthright.

The published version of the autopsy report documented a postmortem examination of Kennedy's remains that was incomplete, confusing, inadequate, and bungled. The causes of such an astonishingly incompetent performance by three military physicians are obscure. It is crystal clear, however, that the three pathologists were under significant duress; they were not free agents in carrying out what was probably the most important autopsy of the century. The minimal standards demanded by the Armed Forces Institute of Pathology for autopsies done by Armed Forces personnel or in Armed Forces facilities were not approached.

The deficiencies in the autopsy as published were so extensive as to preclude the effects of crisis, emotion, bewilderment, or confusion as explanations. The final document was the end result of a planned series of modifications, roadblocks, alterations, and suppressions. Human error may explain some of the deficiencies. To explain them all demands willful actions on the part of persons in unique seats of authority and power.

The President's Clothing

A grave mistake was made, by whose fault is not clear, when the late President's clothing was removed and the body was wrapped in a sheet or sheets. In any homicide case it is elementary and usual that the victim's clothing remain in place. Later the pathologist, as an integral part of his autopsy procedure, removes the clothing from the corpse in an orderly manner.

The clothing was apparently removed by hospital nurses, stuffed into paper bags, and handed to Secret Service Agent William Robert Greer (Hearings, vol. 2, p. 125). When asked whether he saw a hole or tear in the shirt or tie of the late John F. Kennedy, Greer denied seeing such. He admitted that he had not inspected the items very closely because they were in the paper bags.

According to Greer's testimony "two shopping bags" were obtained, and as he held them a nurse stuffed the late President's clothing into the two bags. The items Greer maintained were given to him were: shoes, socks, pants, jacket, shirt, shorts, and body brace. According to Greer there was no undershirt. Greer seemed positive about the matter and under oath volunteered, concerning the late President, "he normally didn't wear an undershirt."

The body brace, according to Greer, was not as large as might be suspected. When quizzed about it by lawyer Arlen Specter, Greer explained. "It looked like . . . a corset-type brace, maybe 6 inches wide, he wore it around . . . his haunches, a little lower than the waist . . . just probably below his belt . . . it was something he normally wore" (Hearings, vol. 2, p. 125). Further, Greer suggested that it was soft, a corsetlike material, possible "elastic."

The clothing was apparently never available to the pathologists who did the autopsy until months after the postmortem examination; they then were given a glimpse of the suit coat and the shirt shortly before they were to testify under oath. Thus, there was no way to check firsthand the alignment of body holes with clothing holes. The wandering nonfatal back wound of the President was a direct outcome of this uninformed and unconventional handling of the murder victim's clothing.

Cleaning of the Corpse

Another nonprofessional endeavor in the face of an obvious homicide was revealed in the testimony of Miss Henchliffe, R.N., of Parkland Memorial Hospital. She and Diana Bowron, R.N., undressed the corpse and in the approved manner for noncriminal deaths cleaned up the body (Hearings, vol. 6, pp. 134, 139). They then wrapped the body in "sheets" and later the corpse was put in a casket.

During the undressing and cleanup procedure, neither nurse apparently observed any wound in the back of the corpse. The back wound seems to have been first observed by the autopsy (Hearings, vol. 2, p. 103). However, a Secret Service agent had seen a shot hit the President's back (Hearings, vol. 2, p. 542).

Supplementary Autopsy Report

Commission Exhibit Number 391 is the supplementary report of the autopsy on the late President John F. Kennedy. It contained general comments about the formalin-fixed brain of the President. It also carried this statement. "In the interest of preserving the specimen coronal sections are not made." Specifically, the pathologists admitted that the brain was not routinely and properly dissected (as all gunshot wounds to the head demand) by slicing it carefully into thin sections to reveal hidden bullet fragments and to demonstrate tracks of bullets and bullet fragments. What in the world the brain was being saved for is not apparent. Its sole value was and is (if it still exists and has not been destroyed or permitted to deteriorate) to reveal more information of a critical nature about the characteristics of the head wound that killed John F. Kennedy.

A listing of tissues that were sampled for microscopic examination was given in this supplement. Brief descriptions of the microscopic sections of the following organs were given: brain at torn edges, heart, lungs, liver, spleen, kidneys, and skin wounds. No mention was made of endocrine organs such as thyroid or adrenals. No reference was made to sections from the anterior throat wound (skin or tracheal cartilages). Apparently no bone was taken from the edges of the bullet entry hole in the back of the head.

The skin wounds mentioned were confusing. "Sections through wounds in the occipital and upper right posterior thoracic regions are essentially similar." Note the admission that the wound in the back of the President's body was in the thoracic (chest) region, not the cervical (neck) region. How could a section through the scalp at the back of the head be "essentially" similar to a section through the hairless skin of the posterior thorax? A beginning histology student knows differently.

No mention was made of signs of putrefaction or autolysis in the various tissue sections at the cellular level. The President was pronounced legally dead about 1:00 PM Dallas time. The President's remains were logged into Bethesda Naval Hospital at about 7:35 PM 22 November 1963. According to the Report, "X-rays and photographs were taken preliminarily and the pathological examination began at about 8 p.m." EST (Report, p. 59). The autopsy was concluded at about 11:00 PM (Report, p. 60).

At 1:00 PM in the heat of Dallas, the remains had been put into a casket; no mention of embalming or refrigeration was made. The dead body was transported from Texas to Maryland. Tissue samples were not fixed any earlier than the time the autopsy began, i.e. about 8:00 PM. It is strange that all the sections were "normal" and that none showed cellular signs of decomposition. Liver and lung are prone to break down relatively quickly after death; spleen also does not resist decomposition. In the supplemental report the liver sections showed well-preserved normal cell structure. Lung and kidney sections showed nothing remarkable.

Perhaps the slides were read in a cursory fashion. In a case of national, indeed international, significance it would be expected that vigorous professional efforts be devoted to making all examinations as thorough as possible.

Perhaps any significant details were edited out of the supplement before it reached the printer. The final paragraph of the basic autopsy report stated, "A supplementary report will be submitted following more detailed examination of the brain and of microscopic section. However, it is not anticipated that these examinations will materially alter the findings" (Report, p. 543). Such a statement is not in the best of scientific tradition. One should not make up one's mind and formulate final conclusions until *all* the data are collected and evaluated.

It must be clearly realized that failure to dissect the brain is beyond comprehension. It is so out of keeping with the practice of even a general pathologist that its omission in a murder case of national importance makes it virtually certain that the pathologists were prevented from making such an examination, or that they made the examination and a report on it but the printed version is a completely fictitious creation.

The Validity of the Autopsy Report

The validity of the printed findings of the John F. Kennedy postmortem examination has been open to serious challenge, and rightly so, from the time of publication of the document.

The inability of the pathologists to find evidence of perforation of the inner chest wall by drainage tubes inserted before death by skilled surgeons raises questions about the surgeons or the pathologists.

Either the emergency room surgeons botched a routine lifesaving procedure or the autopsy pathologists were less than thorough. Were photographs taken of the interior of the chest cavity? Were they clear enough to show details of the entire inner lining of the chest wall? Why was this discrepancy not resolved by a medical conference among the emergency room surgeons and the autopsy pathologists, excluding from the deliberations all persons who did not have firsthand information relevant to the solution? It seems strange that the Warren Commission, which was created for the specific purpose of clarifying the entire matter of the murder of President John F. Kennedy, did not insure such a conference before the various medical experts were asked to testify. Perhaps the Commission was so bewitched by the adversary trial-like scenario they were creating that they could not visualize more effective ways of getting at the truth.

The peculiar flaplike wound of the scalp on the left rear part of the President's head was not mentioned in the autopsy report. A careful examination of the twenty-six volumes of the Warren Commission Hearings and Exhibits revealed a brief reference to the matter by Doctor Marion Jenkins, one of the physicians who attended the moribund President at Parkland Memorial Hospital. Doctor Jenkins observed that when the President was brought into the emergency room, the wound in question was bleeding; this fact demonstrates that it was made before death. It is reasonable to conclude that the flaplike wound was related to the assassination event. Adequate autopsy technique would have insured that a piece of tissue from the border of this wound was taken and examined under the microscope. The wound should also have been traced to ascertain whether the underlying bone was intact. If not, sections from the bone defect should have been evaluated.

Doctor Cyril Wecht, who has examined this photograph of the flaplike wound in the left rear scalp in the National Archives, contends that the wound was too small to have resulted from the passage of a whole bullet. He suggests that this flaplike wound may have resulted from a fragment of a bullet passing out through that portion of the scalp.

This flaplike wound may have had more significance than first met the eye. If the President were shot in the back with a bullet that traveled upward through his throat, and if he were also shot in the head by a bullet coming from the right and the rear as the Warren Commission contended, how could the wound in the left rear of the head *not* raise a number of pertinent questions? It has become even more obvious that the pathologists did not make a thorough search of the President's head to ascertain whether more than one bullet struck him. There is no record that part of the postmortem examination consisted of a routine combing of the head hair to reveal any hidden bullet hole of entrance. The late President had a generous thatch of head hair, a condition conducive to hiding bullet holes of entrance in the scalp if such there were.

The preserved brain is claimed to be missing from the National Archives at this time. If found and studied properly, it might give some information about this odd wound and also about the reported wound of entrance into the left temple region.

Because of the strange and almost nightmarish handling of the autopsy materials by the central government, it is not unreasonable to surmise that the brain contains information which could demand a drastic revision of the published and obviously edited version of the autopsy report. It may be that the resulting changes would require a complete revision of the Warren Commission conclusions.

The administrative maneuvering by the central government officials with respect to the autopsy materials has done much to further distrust of the official conclusions of the Warren Commission. A number of panels have been called to examine portions of the materials. None has been given a free hand. The panels were restricted by the materials given them; the members were selected in such a way as to raise questions of the objectivity of the groups.

For example, sometime Attorney General Ramsey Clark called together a number of medical men to reexamine some of the assassination materials. They came up with an answer that reinforced the government's position; the scientific community was not impressed.

The quality of the selection process in admitting "screened" individuals to see the autopsy materials was best illustrated by the first medical man approved to look at some of the material in custody of the National Archives. He was not a forensic scientist; he was not a pathologist; he was not an expert in crime detection. He was a urologist, an expert in diseases of the kidney, bladder, and associated organs of the human body.

CHAPTER 6

THE PRESIDENTIAL COMMISSION AND ITS CONCLUSIONS

THE makeup of the President's Commission on the assassination of President Kennedy follows.

PRESIDENT'S COMMISSION ON THE ASSASSINATION OF PRESIDENT KENNEDY

CHIEF JUSTICE EARL WARREN, *Chairman*

SENATOR RICHARD B. RUSSELL	REPRESENTATIVE GERALD R. FORD
SENATOR JOHN SHERMAN COOPER	MR. ALLEN W. DULLES
REPRESENTATIVE HALE BOGGS	MR. JOHN J. McCLOY

J. LEE RANKIN, *General Counsel*

Assistant Counsel

FRANCIS W. H. ADAMS	ALBERT E. JENNER, JR.
JOSEPH A. BALL	WESLEY J. LIEBELER
DAVID W. BELIN	NORMAN REDLICH
WILLIAM T. COLEMAN, JR.	W. DAVID SLAWSON
MELVIN ARON EISENBERG	ARLEN SPECTER
BURT W. GRIFFIN	SAMUEL A. STERN
LEON D. HUBERT, JR.	HOWARD P. WILLENS*

Staff Members
PHILLIP BARSON
EDWARD A. CONROY
JOHN HART ELY
ALFRED GOLDBERG
MURRAY J. LAULICHT
ARTHUR MARMOR
RICHARD M. MOSK
JOHN J. O'BRIEN

---

*Mr. Willens also acted as liaison between the Commission and the Department of Justice.

STUART POLLAK
ALFREDDA SCOBEY
CHARLES N. SHAFFER, JR.
LLOYD L. WEINREB

It is important to recognize that "Commission hearings were closed to the public unless the witness appearing before the Commission requested an open hearing" (Report, p. xiii). Apparently only one witness requested an open hearing. Thus, the smog of secrecy has infected the official investigation from the very beginning.

In the Report it is maintained that "the Commission is committing all of its reports and working papers to the National Archives, where they can be permanently preserved under the rules and regulations of the National Archives and applicable Federal law" (Report, p. xv). The statement fails to add " . . . and in deference to the whims of the Kennedy dynasty lawyers." Perhaps the careful wording of this statement needs examination, e.g. the "reports" and "working papers" of the Commission were filed in the Archives. Does this assertion mean that critical *materials* were not part of this file? Could it be that, cynically, the Commission excluded the critical items of the case from their file, e.g. autopsy materials (brain, tissue sections), detailed unaltered draft of autopsy report, x-rays, and photographs taken at autopsy?

There is reason to maintain that the Commission indeed may have performed such a sleight-of-hand maneuver. Hence, scholars must go hat in hand, pulling the forelock, to the Kennedy dynasty lawyers for permission to examine the most important materials associated with the crime, the autopsy samples themselves, the x-rays of the remains, and the photographs said to have been taken during the autopsy.

The situation is unprecedented in a nation that pretends to be governed by laws not by men.

The National Archives

An interesting but strange aspect of the custodial attitudes demonstrated by the National Archives personnel is told by Thompson (1976). He wished to establish directly the weight of the pristine bullet (Commission Exhibit No. 399) found at Parkland Hospital and compare the weight with that of two test rounds fired into cotton waste (Commission Exhibit No. 572). He therefore carried a sensitive balance (Mettler® brand, which is highly thought of by scientists) to the National Archives in order to make precise weighings. Thompson reported " . . . The Deputy Archivist denied permission for these bullets to be weighed." The weighing process is harmless and not destructive to the items weighed.

Executive Sessions

Recently, the transcripts of a number of executive sessions of the Commission were made available after years of being suppressed. These documents revealed for the first time some surprising aspects of the Commission and its competence (*New Republic*, 1975).

The Commission meeting on 6 December 1963 revealed the uninformed attitude of its members concerning the importance of forensic science data in arriving at a sound conclusion.

Senator Cooper, Mr. McCloy, and Chairman Warren all expressed confusion over the matter of the bullets and where they went. Senator Russell complained, "They couldn't find where one bullet came out that struck the President and yet they found a bullet in the stretcher."

McCloy suggested that the Commission should have the autopsy documents available — hardly an earthshattering suggestion. Warren thought it a good idea, especially since the FBI reports were so foggy and unsatisfactory. A regular theme of dissatisfaction over the FBI and its inability to generate meaningful and useful reports for the Commission was evident.

It is difficult to understand how the Commission was confused over the *crucial* role of a competent autopsy report in the evaluation of a gunshot homicide.

The Chief Justice of the nation's Supreme Court could not plead ignorance; he was involved in decisions of law involving every aspect of adequate legal proof. It is obvious that, assuming his mental competence at the time of the Commission operations, he knew full well the essential nature of hard evidence in a homicide case. The irony of the situation was that, in all probability, had a homicide conviction been appealed to the Supreme Court on the basis of evidence having the qualities that the Warren Commission accepted and indeed forced, the Warren Court would have thrown out the conviction.

One or two of the staff lawyers for the Commission seemed to have reasonably sound legal qualifications — sound enough at least to know the critical blunder being perpetrated in the Commission's refusal to examine the pertinent medicolegal evidence and in refusing access to that evidence by the very pathologists who generated some of it.

A memorandum from Arlen Specter 30 April 1964 to J. Lee Rankin, Chief Council for the Commission, expressed concern for the lack of access to the photographs and x-rays of John F. Kennedy's autopsy. He wrote in the memo, "the Commission should determine with certainty whether the shots came from the rear."

Specter also admitted that the surgeons who rendered aid to the stricken President at Parkland Memorial Hospital had not observed the President's back nor the hole in the back of his head.

Nevertheless, the only truly relevant materials in the case (the complete autopsy findings and exhibits) were ignored by the Commission and its staff.

The Autopsy Personnel

Autopsies under military control are to be attended only by personnel contributing to the scientific examination of the remains. Others are to be excluded. Was that directive observed in the autopsy of John F. Kennedy's corpse?

According to FBI observers at the autopsy, Special Agents O'Neill and Sibert of the FBI and Secret Service Agents Roy Kellerman, William Greer, and William O'Leary "were the only personnel other than medical personnel present during the autopsy." Later in the FBI report, nonmedical personnel in addition to these were said to have been present.

The complete list of those attending the autopsy according to O'Neill and Sibert follows.

1. Admiral C.B. Holloway, U.S.N. Commanding Officer, U.S. Naval Medical Center, Bethesda, Maryland.
2. Admiral Berkley [*sic*] U.S.N., President's personal physician.
3. Commander James J. Humes, Chief Pathologist, Bethesda Naval Hospital, conducted autopsy.
4. Captain James H. Stoner, Jr., Commanding Officer, U.S. Naval Medical School, Bethesda, Maryland.
5. Mr. John T. Stringer, Jr., medical photographer.
6. Brigadier General Godfrey McHugh, the President's Air Force Military Aide (another nonmedical general who might have forbidden the pathologists to dissect the throat wound?).
7. Doctor George Bakeman.

The roles played by most of the persons listed in execution of the autopsy on President John F. Kennedy's remains are not apparent.

It was clear, too, that some Commission members were impressed with the importance of getting a deposition from the late President's widow as soon as possible. They realized that she was closest to him when the bullets struck.

In the Commission meeting of 21 January 1964 there was evident perplexity over the President's wounds. McCloy asked why the FBI report gave a version of the wounds not in accord with the much delayed (and obviously much edited) autopsy report. The bewilderment of the Commission members raises the question of why they did not hire their own forensic science experts to advise and interpret technical data for them.

Doubts on the part of Commission members as to the accuracy of FBI reports and FBI responses to queries and challenges were obvious during these secret meetings. There was also clear evidence that the Commission members were literally terrified at the prospect of offending J. Edgar Hoover. The situation was such as to make a reasonably thorough probe of the many critical aspects of the J.F. Kennedy murder virtually impossible.

During a discussion of how to disprove that Oswald was an informer for the FBI, the CIA, or both, Allan Dulles admitted such proof to be well-nigh impossible because key personnel in those agencies would lie even under oath to prevent "embarassment" to their respective agencies.

Another difficulty is apparent as a result of this secret meeting: Dulles misled the Commission with respect to domestic activities of the CIA. Dulles' role in the Commission's deliberations remains obscure but disquieting.

At this meeting, the question of J.F. Kennedy's wounds was introduced by Rankin. The question of whether the wound in the front of the neck was an entrance or exit wound came up. Rankin recognized the contradictions between the reports from doctors at Parkland Memorial Hospital and the autopsy version made available to the Commission. Rankin realized that a basic problem in their investigation was the specific nature of the anterior neck wound.

Rankin also expressed the Commission's confusion about the pristine bullet found under odd circumstances in Parkland Hospital. The conflicting testimony about the bullet was clearly revealed in this meeting.

The Unidentified Photograph

An executive session was held by the Warren Commission on 27 January 1964 at which Rankin made a summation of the evidence concerning the back wound in the President's remains. He was reported as saying, "We have an explanation here in the autopsy that probably a fragment came out the front of the neck, but with the elevation the shot must have come from, and the angle, it seems quite apparent now, since we have the picture of where the bullet entered in the back, that the bullet entered below the shoulder blades to the right of the backbone, which is below the place where the picture shows the bullet came out in the neckband of the shirt in front. . . ."

Several points are of interest in this statement. First, the

Commission had some sort of unidentified photograph, presumably of Kennedy's back wound. The location of the wound was said to be in the thoracic (chest) region, not in the neck. Rankin was understandably bewildered at how a bullet on a downward angle could enter the body in the chest region and exit from the anterior throat at the level of about the third tracheal ring, especially if no bones were struck to cause a deflection of the bullet as it traversed the body.

The version of the autopsy report published in the final Warren Commission Report asserted that the bullet that entered the President's back exited from the anterior throat. Unfortunately, the official published version of the autopsy report was not dated.

Secondly, the unidentified photograph was said to show the bullet hole located in the back *below* the shoulder blades, a location more in accord with published autopsy sketches and bullet holes in the late President's suit coat and shirt than with the official Commission contention of a hole in the lower neck.

In the secret meeting of the Commission on 30 April 1964 the autopsy pictures were discussed. Reports from the Parkland Memorial Hospital doctors, the autopsy physicians at Bethesda Naval Medical Center, and Governor Connally's testimony supported by that of his wife were in conflict with respect to angles of the bullets that were fired. It is not apparent that these conflicts were resolved then nor in the final published report of the Commission.

Rankin rambled on:

> We have a very serious problem in the record . . . that the bullet . . . probably passed through the President and then through Governor Connally. And we now have the testimony of Governor Connally that that could not have happened. He is certain it did not happen. And that the bullet that struck him is one that did not hit the President. We also have some drawings of President Kennedy which are reconstructions by the men that participated in the autopsy. And these men have not seen those pictures of the autopsy, but they had these drawings made, and we do not know whether those drawings conform to the pictures of the autopsy or not. Now, I thought we could avoid having those pictures being a part of

our record, because the family has a strong feeling about them, and I think we should respect it insofar as can possibly be done, and carry out the work of the Commission — because they do not want the President to be remembered in connection with those pictures . . . But I feel that a doctor and some member of the Commission should examine them sufficiently so that they could report to the Commission that there is nothing inconsistent with the other findings in connection with the matter in those pictures. In that way we can avoid any question that we have passed anything up that the Commission should know or that we have not tried to take advantage of information that should be available to us. . . .

It is apparent that Rankin, at least, had an intuitive feeling for the nonsense of the artist's sketches of the bullet tracks in the President's body. Nevertheless, the unvalidated sketches were included in the testimony and, using them as a base, detailed angular measurements were made. The gross incompetence of any group that would be a party to such deceptive and uninformed procedures of investigation strains the mind. Moreover, the concern for the "feelings of the family" was either dissimulation or a more disturbing stance on the part of an official investigator for the people, deferring to a special class, royal family, or dynasty. Evidence in felony cases is not used or suppressed at the whim of the victim's survivors — or is that procedure applicable only to "the great unwashed," the ordinary citizens of the United States? Are there select clans that are above the law?

The Chairman's response to Rankin's concern was " . . . but without putting those pictures in our record. We do not want those in our record . . . It would make it a morbid thing for all time to come . . ."

Death investigations of all sorts have a habit of being morbid. Murder is a morbid event. When murder is inadequately investigated by an official body charged to probe the depths of the incident because of considerations that are incompetent, immaterial, and irrelevant, the finger of shame points at that group; for all time that group (the Warren Commission) will be known for its dereliction.

The comment by the chairman was an emotional one that

reflected a lack of understanding for the elements of scientific proof and legal propriety.

The overall impact of revealing these secret meetings is a sharp demonstration that critical matters were never resolved by the Commission. The uncovering of the truth was *not* the primary concern of the Commission members. Medical evidence was to be buried for the frivolous reason of the "feelings" of the victim's family. Political and administrative considerations seemed to be held of greater importance by the Commission than the uncompromising search for the truth.

Finally, the competence of the Commission to do its job as assigned was revealed to be questionable. The final Report was obviously a compromise of significant proportions made by confused men possessing few qualifications for the task that they undertook (Osborne, 1975; Szulc, 1975; Marshall, 1975).

The Single Bullet Theory

The origin of the single bullet that the Commission postulates went through both Kennedy and Connally and emerged in an undeformed condition, except for the engraving of the rifling on the metal jacket is questionable. The bullet was found by the chief engineer of Parkland Memorial Hospital some time in the afternoon of the day Kennedy was murdered (Report, p. 81). It was further claimed that the engineer Tomlinson found the bullet while he was shifting stretchers about, on and off an elevator (Hearings, vol. 6, pp. 126-131). But Tomlinson denied that the bullet did in fact fall off the stretcher used for Connally; apparently it came from another stretcher of unknown origin, but clearly not Connally's (Report, p. 81).

The Report said, "although Tomlinson was not certain whether the bullet came from the Connally stretcher or an adjacent one . . ." The testimony of Tomlinson was a bit stronger than that; it reflected more nearly a denial that the bullet came from the Connally stretcher rather than his being "not certain." The Commission, ignoring part of Tomlinson's testimony, decided that the bullet came from Connally's stretcher. The argument was strange; "evidence which elimi-

nated President Kennedy's stretcher as a source of the bullet"
was used to prove that it came from Connally's stretcher, although a number of other stretchers were about the hospital
and in the immediate vicinity (Report, p. 81).

From the rigid evidential point of view, Commission Exhibit
Number 399 has no value. It is a bullet that, according to FBI
tests, was once fired through the alleged murder rifle. No con-
nection of any acceptable sort has been made between the bullet
(Exhibit No. 399) and the actual event, the murder of a man,
John F. Kennedy, who was at the time President of the United
States.

Conspiracy

The conclusions of the Commission as published in the official Report were carefully worded and do not always mean
exactly what they appear to say on the surface. For example,
"The Commission has found no evidence that either Lee
Harvey Oswald or Jack Ruby was part of any conspiracy, domestic or foreign, to assassinate President Kennedy." "No evidence was found" left a door or two open to the possibility that
such evidence might exist and might be found later; the door
has not been slammed shut on the possibility that the Commission did not follow through on certain routes of evidence (Report, p. 21).

Another interesting statement was made (Report, p. 22). "On
the basis of the evidence before the Commission it concludes
that Oswald acted alone." The phrase "the evidence before the
Commission," when used by a covey of lawyers, was a quali-
fying phrase with all kinds of possibilities. Did the disclaimer
reveal an uncertainty or feeling of discomfort on the part of the
Commission with respect to its conclusions? Was there in fact
other evidence (now held in strange secrecy by the National
Archives) available to the Commission and known to exist by at
least some of its members but not *formally* brought before the
Commission? Was there other evidence in addition to the suppressed autopsy photographs positively deleted from consideration by the Commission and thus not "evidence before the

Commission"?

One statement in the official conclusion seemed strong and unequivocal. "In its entire investigation the Commission has found no evidence of conspiracy, subversion, or disloyalty to the U.S. Government by any Federal, State, or local official" (Report, p. 22). If "entire investigation" meant what it seems to, then there can be nothing in the secret files at the Archives that would modify that conclusion. Minutes of several executive sessions of the Commission seemed to suggest that all members of the Commission, at one time at least, were not comfortable with the reports obtained from the Federal Bureau of Investigation and the Central Intelligence Agency. It would also be appropriate to conclude that there was nothing in the suppressed medicolegal evidence that would put into question the conclusion of the Commission about official loyalty. Thus, one is again perplexed by the compulsive drive to hide materials from probing by scholars.

Perhaps the Commission's definition of disloyalty did not include the substantial alteration by Naval officers of high rank of an official autopsy report in defiance of Armed Forces directives on the details of an adequate medicolegal autopsy.

Dissimulation

A claim was made in the Report that if not false, was at least deceitful (p. 1970). "The wounds of entry and exit on the President were approximated based on information gained from the autopsy reports and photographs." In the Hearings it was made clear that not even the autopsy pathologists were permitted to see the photographs allegedly made at the autopsy. No reason was given. The published record of the Warren Commission gave the lie to this claim. One wonders why the claim was made.

The conclusion concerning the angle of the shot that struck the President in the back at the level of the third thoracic vertebra was that "the probable angle through the President's body was calculated at 17° 43′ 30″, assuming he was sitting in a vertical position" (Report, p. 106). Photographs taken the instant before the President was shot showed him sitting in an upright position held there by his body brace.

It is apparent that the writer of the Report was aware of the questionable nature of the statement made about the angle of the shots. The second paragraph on page 107 of the Report hedges on the shot angles in such a way as to destroy these measurements as meaningful data. "Governor Connally's doctors measured an angle of declination on his body from the entry wound on his back to the exit on the front of his chest at about 25° when he sat erect" (Report, p. 107).

The lining up of the 17 to 18 degree downward path of the single bullet through Kennedy with the 25 degree downward path of the bullet that went through Connally was a feat of legerdemain. The lateral line-up of these wounds cannot be accomplished so that a single bullet makes both wounds without involving two right-angle turns in midair by any alleged single bullet.

According to the Report (p. 110), the President was 265.3 feet from the alleged murder rifle when he was struck in the head by a bullet said to have come from the sixth floor window of the Texas School Book Depository Building at a downward angle of 15 degrees 21 minutes.

The value of these "precise" angular measurements is unclear with the exception of the wound track through Connally. The angular path of a bullet through the body of the victim is of basic importance. Calculated angles based on hypothetical locations, speeds, and elevations have little value unless confirmed by autopsy data.

The Commission, probably because it totally lacked any competence in forensic science, worked backwards in evaluating the incident. The facts of the shooting as revealed in the remains of the President and in Connally's wounds are given; they are not arguable. Other observations, calculations, and hypotheses must be squared with what the victim's body indicated, not the other way around.

For example, if extension backward of the 25 degree downward bullet track through Connally led to some point other than the supposed firing position of the Commission's killer candidate, it would be clear that the location of the shooter must be changed. It is unwarranted to decide where the killer had to have been (for whatever reason) and then attempt to explain out of existence medicolegal facts that were not in accord with the predetermined conclusion.

The Commission and Adversary System*

There is an uneasy relationship of long standing between expert witnesses and trial lawyers. The latter dislike and do not fully understand the experts. The experts in turn find it increasingly difficult to function in an acceptable manner under the adversary system as it is practiced in American law.

Nowhere is this tense relationship better illustrated than in the testimony of the various "experts" called by the lawyers on the staff of the Warren Commission.

The record of the Hearings amply illustrated the lawyers' concern, not for the whole truth, but only for the pieces of truth that would support the preconceived "case" formulated by the staff of the Commission. It is clear from the Hearings that the adversary format is *uniquely unfit* for use in group investigations aimed at digging out all the truth. The history of the Hearings bears ample testimony to the fact that, had the Commission members been competent and had all the facts been explored, the truth still would not have been brought to the surface because the adversary format is designed not to disclose the truth, but rather to help one side or the other win a fight.

The discomfort of such experts as the physicians from Park-

---

*An explanation for the peculiar adversary approach used by the Warren Commission lawyers in their presumed pursuit of the truth of the assassination may rest in the contention of Chief Justice Warren that the proceedings were in fact a "trial" (Hearings, vol. 1, p. 128). Because the Chief Justice set the theme, it was unfortunate that no meaningful and effective effort was made to insure cross-examination by counsel taking an adversary position to the Commission staff lawyers. The appointment of Walter E. Craig, then president of the American Bar Association, to represent Oswald (deceased) and his family was cynical tokenism. Craig's participation was of such magnitude that he was referred to once in the Report and his name can be found nowhere in the Index to the official Report.

land Hospital who had treated the moribund President was clearly revealed during their testimony. The atmosphere of the Hearings can be best appreciated by reading the testimony of Doctor Perry. The doctors were bullied; they were made to feel that they were on trial for something or other; they were so interrogated as to have their direct testimony twisted, curtailed, and otherwise manipulated so that it fit into the "case" to be won by the staff lawyers.

In various places where expert testimony was impregnable against the adversary attacks of the Commission staff lawyers, that testimony was simply ignored; indeed in some places the testimony was misstated in the "summation" of the Commission "case" as printed in the Report volume.

In courtroom experience as an expert witness, the author has too often found himself being villified and shoved into a quasi-"on trial" position by the opposing attorney during the testimony in order to destroy the value of some technical data or procedure. There is a cynicism among lawyers in this matter; one week a prosecutor tears apart an expert and his data when the defense presents it. The next trial may find that same prosecutor using similar data and technical procedures to support his prosecution. It is no wonder that the expert is as bewildered as the public.

For the technical expert who attempts to advise the court, the situation approaches the intolerable. Under the present adversary conditions there is serious doubt whether the required oath to tell the truth, the *whole truth,* and nothing but the truth can in most instances be observed. The adversary lawyers control the proceedings. The last thing they want is that part of the "whole truth" that might weaken their respective cases.

The results of the endeavors of the Warren Commission are a strong indictment of the adversary system for the manner in which it compromises expert testimony in American courts. The critical need for drastic changes in the handling of expert testimony by American courts is obvious to numerous experts.

Recently a number of books that purport to present facts as they occurred have appeared dealing with aspects of the John F. Kennedy murder. For example, Morrow (1976) has had published what he claims to be a reconstruction of clandestine events that were integral parts of the Kennedy assassination. If this book is indeed factual and nonfictional, its implications are devastating to our central government.

The author is reputed to have been a former CIA employee (operative, agent, consultant; Who knows what name to give him?). Certain technical errors and impossible "facts" make the book suspect as nonfiction. The point is clear however; had the Warren Commission carried out an honest, competent, and forthright investigation, much of the Kennedy murder mythology would have been forestalled. The fact that lies (even "white lies") by government agencies spawn bigger and more malignant lies is apparently unrecognized by the current (1977) House Select Committee on Assassinations.

CHAPTER 7

CRITIQUE:
THE RIFLE AND CARTRIDGES

MUCH controversy has surrounded the quality of the rifle used in the murder of John F. Kennedy. The Warren Commission judged it adequate to do the job as they concluded it was done.*

Robert Frazier was an FBI firearms expert who tested the Mannlicher-Carcano rifle alleged to have been used in the murder. His fastest time for firing three shots in a row was 4.6 seconds. He testified that in order to do so the gun was fired as fast as he could operate the bolt, (Hearings, vol. 3, p. 407) without regard for accuracy.

Because there is such divided opinion concerning the rifle used in the murder and the cartridges, it seems appropriate to include verbatim just what the Commission published about the matter.

Expert Examination of Rifle, Cartridge Cases, and Bullet Fragments

On the sixth floor of the Depository Building, the Dallas police found three spent cartridges and a rifle. A nearly whole bullet was discovered in the stretcher used to carry Governor Connally at Parkland Hospital. As described in the preceding section, five bullet fragments were found in the President's limousine. The cartridge cases, the nearly whole bullet and the bullet fragments were all subjected to firearms identification analysis by qualified experts. It was the unanimous

---

*Meunier (1976) has reviewed the problems surrounding the rifle, the empty 6.5 mm rifle cartridge cases discovered, and Commission Exhibit Number 399 (the so-called mysterious, undeformed bullet that was essential to the one bullet theory of the Commission). He showed clearly how the Warren Commission's evaluation of the alleged murder weapon, ammunition, and Oswald's shooting ability was incompetent.

opinion of the experts that the nearly whole bullet, the two largest bullet fragments and the three cartridge cases were definitely fired in the rifle found on the sixth floor of the Depository Building to the exclusion of all other weapons.

Discovery of Cartridge Cases and Rifle

Shortly after the assassination, police officers arrived at the Depository Building and began a search for the assassin and evidence. Around 1 p.m. Deputy Sheriff Luke Mooney noticed a pile of cartons in front of the window in the southeast corner of the sixth floor. (See Commission Exhibit No. 723, p. 80) Searching that area he found at approximately 1:12 p.m. three empty cartridge cases on the floor near the window. When he was notified of Mooney's discovery, Capt. J. W. Fritz, chief of the homicide bureau of the Dallas Police Department, issued instructions that nothing be moved or touched until technicians from the police crime laboratory could take photographs and check for fingerprints. Mooney stood guard to see that nothing was disturbed. A few minutes later, Lt. J. C. Day of the Dallas Police Department arrived and took photographs of the cartridge cases before anything had been moved.

At 1:22 p.m. Deputy Sheriff Eugene Boone and Deputy Constable Seymour Weitzman found a bolt-action rifle with a telescopic sight between two rows of boxes in the northwest corner near the staircase on the sixth floor. No one touched the weapon or otherwise disturbed the scene until Captain Fritz and Lieutenant Day arrived and the weapon was photographed as it lay on the floor. After Lieutenant Day determined that there were no fingerprints on the knob of the bolt and that the wooden stock was too rough to take fingerprints, he picked the rifle up by the stock and held it that way while Captain Fritz opened the bolt and ejected a live round. Lieutenant Day retained possession of the weapon and took it back to the police department for examination. Neither Boone nor Weitzman handled the rifle.

Discovery of Bullet at Parkland Hospital

A nearly whole bullet was found on Governor Connally's

stretcher at Parkland Hospital after the assassination. After his arrival at the hospital the Governor was brought into trauma room No. 2 on a stretcher, removed from the room on that stretcher a short time later, and taken on an elevator to the second-floor operating room. On the second floor he was transferred from the stretcher to an operating table which was then moved into the operating room, and a hospital attendant wheeled the empty stretcher into an elevator. Shortly afterward, Darrell C. Tomlinson, the hospital's senior engineer, removed this stretcher from the elevator and placed it in the corridor on the ground floor, alongside another stretcher wholly unconnected with the care of Governor Connally. A few minutes later, he bumped one of the stretchers against the wall and a bullet rolled out.

Although Tomlinson was not certain whether the bullet came from the Connally stretcher or the adjacent one, the Commission has concluded that the bullet came from the Governor's stretcher. The conclusion is buttressed by evidence which eliminated President Kennedy's stretcher as a source of the bullet. President Kennedy remained on the stretcher on which he was carried into the hospital while the doctors tried to save his life. He was never removed from the stretcher from the time he was taken into the emergency room until his body was placed in a casket in that same room. After the President's body was removed from that stretcher, the linen was taken off and placed in a hamper and the stretcher was pushed into trauma room No. 2, a completely different location from the site where the nearly whole bullet was found.

Description of Rifle

The bolt-action, clip-fed rifle found on the sixth floor of the Depository, described more fully in appendix X, is inscribed with various markings, including "MADE ITALY," "CAL. 6.5," "1940" and the number C2766. (See Commission Exhibit Nos. 1303, 541(2) and 541(3), pp. 82-83). These markings have been explained as follows: "MADE ITALY" refers to its origin; "CAL. 6.5" refers to the rifle's caliber; "1940" refers to the year of manufacture; and the number C2766 is the serial number. This rifle is the only one of its type bearing that serial number.* After review of standard reference works and the markings on the rifle, it was identified by the FBI as a 6.5-millimeter model 91/38 Mannlicher-Carcano rifle. Experts from the FBI made an independent determination of the caliber by inserting a Mannlicher-Carcano 6.5-millimeter cartridge into the weapon for fit, and by making a sulfur cast of the inside of the weapon's barrel and measuring the cast with a micrometer. From outward appearance, the weapon would appear to be a 7.35-millimeter rifle, but its mechanism had been rebarreled with a 6.5-millimeter barrel. Constable Deputy Sheriff Weitzman, who only saw the rifle at a glance and did not handle it, thought the weapon looked like a 7.65 Mauser bolt-action rifle.

The rifle is 40.2 inches long and weighs 8 pounds. The minimum length broken down is 34.8 inches, the length of the wooden stock. (See Commission Exhibit No. 1304, p. 132.) Attached to the weapon is an inexpensive four-power telescopic sight, stamped "Optics Ordnance Inc./Hollywood, California," and "Made in Japan." The weapon also bears a sling consisting of two leather straps. The sling is not a standard rifle sling but appears to be a musical instrument strap or a sling from a carrying case or camera bag.

Expert Testimony

Four experts in the field of firearms identification analyzed the nearly whole bullet, the two largest fragments and the three cartridge cases to determine whether they had been fired from the C2766 Mannlicher-Carcano rifle found on the sixth floor of the Depository. Two of these experts testified before the Commission. One was Robert A. Frazier, a special agent of the FBI assigned to the FBI Laboratory in Washington, D.C. Frazier has worked generally in the field of firearms identification for 23 years, examining firearms of various types for purpose of identifying the caliber and other characteristics of the weapons and making comparisons of bullets and cartridge cases for the purpose of determining whether or not they were fired in a particular weapon. He estimated that he has made "in the neighborhood of 50,000 to 60,000" fire-

---

*This statement is not accurate. As will be explained later, the serial numbering of Italian rifles tended to be rather casual and numbers are known to appear in duplicate and triplicate. (C.G.W.)

arms comparisons and has testified in court on about 400 occasions. The second witness who testified on this subject was Joseph D. Nicol, superintendent of the bureau of criminal identification and investigation for the State of Illinois. Nicol also has had long and substantial experience since 1941 in firearms identification, and estimated that he had made thousands of bullet and cartridge case examinations.

In examining the bullet fragments and cartridge cases, these experts applied the general principles accepted in the field of firearms identification, which are discussed in more detail in appendix X at pages 547-553. In brief, a determination that a particular bullet or cartridge case has been fired in a particular weapon is based upon a comparison of the bullet or case under examination with one or more bullets or cases known to have been fired in that weapon. When a bullet is fired in any given weapon, it is engraved with the characteristics of the weapon. In addition to the rifling characteristics of the barrel which are common to all weapons of a given make and model, every weapon bears distinctive microscopic markings on its barrel, firing pin and bolt face. These markings arise initially during manufacture, since the action of the manufacturing tools differs microscopically from weapon to weapon and since, in addition, the tools change microscopically while being used. As a weapon is used further distinctive markings are introduced. Under microscopic examination a qualified expert may be able to determine whether the markings on a bullet known to have been fired in a particular weapon and the markings on a suspect bullet are the same and, therefore, whether both bullets were fired in the same weapon to the exclusion of all other weapons. Similarly, firearms identification experts are able to compare the markings left upon the base of cartridge cases and thereby determine whether both cartridges were fired by the same weapon to the exclusion of all other weapons. According to Frazier, such an identification "is made on the presence of sufficient individual microscopic characteristics so that a very definite pattern is formed and visualized on the two surfaces." Under some circumstances, as where the bullet or cartridge case is seriously mutilated, there are not sufficient individual characteristics to enable the expert to make a firm identification.

After making independent examinations, both Frazier and

Nicol positively identified the nearly whole bullet from the stretcher and the two larger bullet fragments found in the Presidential limousine as having been fired in the C2766 Mannlicher-Carcano rifle found in the Depository to the exclusion of all other weapons. Each of the two bullet fragments had sufficient unmutilated area to provide the basis for an identification. However, it was not possible to determine whether the two bullet fragments were from the same bullet or from two different bullets. With regard to the other bullet fragments discovered in the limousine and in the course of treating President Kennedy and Governor Connally, however, expert examination could demonstrate only that the fragments were "similar in metallic composition" to each other, to the two larger fragments and to the nearly whole bullet. After examination of the three cartridge cases found on the sixth floor of the Depository, Frazier and Nicol concluded that they had been fired in the C2766 Mannlicher-Carcano rifle to the exclusion of all other weapons. Two other experts from the Federal Bureau of Investigation, who made independent examinations of the nearly whole bullet, bullet fragments and cartridge cases, reached the identical conclusions.

The Rifle

The 6.5 millimeter Mannlicher-Carcano rifle was one of the variants of the model 1891 Mannlicher-Carcano rifle used by the Italian Army; another variant was a 7.35 millimeter piece. It is clear from the evidence available that the Italian Army in World War II was the poorest armed, with respect to rifles, of any of the major powers. The Mannlicher-Carcano rifle is a modification of the Mauser; the Italian rifle is also known as the Mauser Paravicino. The rifle differs from the basic Mauser in that the handle of the bolt sits anterior to the receiver bridge when in the locked position. The outrageous stories about the safety of the rifle may be exaggerations. There is reason to be concerned about reports of the firing pin moving backward toward the shooter in some instances. The accuracy of the rifle would not recommend it as anything but a general issue weapon to put in the hands of mobs of soldiers who are not expert target shooters at best.

In 1940 the Italian government standardized the bore of all its military rifles at 6.5 mm; after that date all Italian military rifles were manufactured in the 6.5 mm version.

The rifle that was claimed to have been used in the murder of John F. Kennedy was a model 1938 6.5 millimeter (91/38) serial number C2766, manufactured in 1940 at the Italian arsenal located at Terni; it was one of a shipment of war surplus Italian rifles sold in the United States. The specifications of rifles of that model were as follows: caliber 6.5 mm; length overall, 40.2 inches; length of barrel, 20.9 inches; front sight, barleycorn; rear sight, fixed; weight, 7.6 pounds; stated muzzle velocity, 2320 feet per second. A six-round nondetachable box magazine was part of this model. Essentially this model was a 6.5 mm modification of the 7.35 mm rifle 1938 model manufactured after the beginning of the second World War.

Serial numbers on these rifles may be misleading. There is information that suggests multiple use of a given serial number. Apparently some foreign governments are not so demanding concerning firearm serial numbers as is true of the

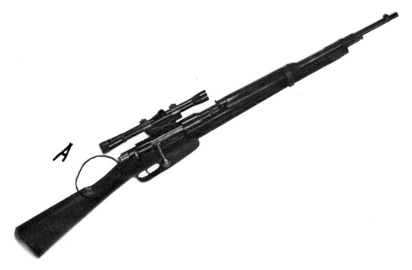

Figure 7-1. This is a photograph of Commission Exhibit Number 747. It shows the rifle C2766 (Hearings, vol. 17, p. 522). It gives a general view of the alleged assassination rifle.

United States government (Smith, 1969).

A report from the FBI to the Warren Commission admitted the questionable value of Italian arsenal serial numbers in the identification of a specific rifle. In the Commission Exhibit Number 2562 it was reported that Mussolini ordered all arms factories in Italy to manufacture the Mannlicher-Carcano rifle. The report then says, "Since many concerns were manufacturing the same weapon, the same serial number appears on weapons manufactured by more than one concern. Some bear a letter prefix and some do not." It is clear that the Warren Commission claim that the weapon found on the sixth floor of the Texas Book Depository Building can be exclusively identified by serial number is not true; the FBI report unequivocally showed that there are probably several such rifles with the identical serial numbers. The serial numbers were just not exclusive.

A perplexing report, which has never been explained adequately in the official investigation, had it that the murder rifle was a 7.65 mm Mauser of German (not Italian) make. This rifle was shown once on national television as the murder gun. It then disappeared in a strange fashion. Perhaps the report was the result of honest confusion and faulty recognition; if so that fact should have been clarified.

The original report apparently came over KBOX, a Dallas television station. The rifle, according to Commission Exhibit Number 3048, was a 7.65 Mauser fitted with a German-manufactured telescopic sight. It was reported to have been found on the staircase at the fifth floor of the Texas Book Depository Building.

Who identified this Mauser rifle?

District Attorney Henry Wade of Dallas maintained that the rifle was a Mauser, according to Commission Exhibit Number 2169.

Deputy Constable Seymour Weitzman, within twenty-four hours of the shooting as indicated in the Commission Exhibit Number 2003, page 63, filed an affidavit with the Dallas police to the effect that he in the company of Deputy Sheriff Boone discovered the rifle in question during a search of the sixth floor of the Book Depository. A quote from the Commission Exhibit Number 2003 is revealing. "This rifle was a 7.65 Mauser bolt action equipped with a thick leather brownish-black sling on it."

Deputy Sheriff Eugene Boone later testified under oath before the Presidential Commission that a Captain Fritz, after close examination of the rifle at the scene, identified the gun as a 7.65 mm Mauser. In written reports, Boone twice informed Sheriff Decker that the rifle was a 7.65 mm Mauser fitted with a scope sight.

The identity of the rifle that was actually found on the sixth floor of the Texas Book Depository Building is still confused. Deputy Sheriff Seymour Weitzman discovered the rifle no longer than sixty minutes after the shooting. He described it as a 7.65 millimeter German Mauser (Commission Exhibit No. 2003, p. 63). A fellow police officer confirmed the identification. Deputy Sheriff Roger D. Craig was present during the search and agreed that the rifle discovered was a Mauser. Craig was reported to have asserted in a letter dated 17 March 1975 that he and Deputy Boone found the rifle. Moreover, he declared that the designation 7.65 Mauser was stamped on the barrel (Anson, 1975).

Deputy Weitzman had previously been manager of a sporting goods store (Hearings, vol. 7, p. 108) and was known to have been widely familiar with firearms. The alleged murder rifle was clearly marked (stamped on the barrel) with the notice "MADE IN ITALY" and the bore "CAL. 6.5" (Hearings, vol. 5, pp. 560-561).

The remembrance of numerous persons of a report, via radio and television, shortly after the President's death that a German Mauser rifle has been found in the Book Depository Building and was of caliber 7.65 mm was given no serious consideration by the Commission. Files of old network radiotapes and videotapes seem to have disappeared or may never have existed. Thus it is almost impossible to track down that memory and evaluate it.

When all the facts that are known fall together, there is strong reason to ask whether two rifles were not in fact found in the Texas Book Depository Building. Was one of the rifles later suppressed for some reason or other?

What subsequently happened to this Mauser rifle? How did the confusion arise? Was a substitution of guns made twenty-four hours after the shooting? These are a few questions which have arisen as a result of less than adequate handling of the matter by the Warren Commission. If there were no substitution or other questionable activity associated with the alleged murder rifle, why then was the affair not cleared up in the definitive Report issued by the Commission?

The Alleged Murder Rifle

The rifle officially identified by the Warren Commission as the murder weapon was a 6.5 mm Mannlicher-Carcano Italian-made weapon, fitted with a cheap telescopic sight of Japanese manufacture.

The alleged murder weapon was described by Sebastian Latona (an FBI firearms expert) as a cheap old weapon (Hearings vol. 4, p. 29).

The conclusions of the Warren Commission about the accuracy of the alleged murder weapon and its reliability rested on misunderstandings of the significance of the tests performed for the Commission and on the cavalier neglect of data that did not fit into the official story, which seems to have been outlined even before the Hearings began.

The specific rifle tested by the FBI as the murder weapon was rusty and badly worn, according to Commission Exhibit Number 2974 published by the Commission. Moreover, the sight had been installed for a left-handed shooter; Oswald, the alleged killer, was right-handed.

A fundamental difficulty with the rifle said to have been used in the murder of John F. Kennedy is the fact that the cheap Japanese telescopic sight could not be aligned with the barrel to allow the user to zero in on any target. J. Edgar Hoover stated the difficulty in a letter reproduced in volume 26 of the Hearings, page 104. The competence of the Commission on rifle matters was illustrated by their conclusion that the defective telescopic sight arrangement would have actually improved the shooter's accuracy, a viewpoint that is unusual among sport shooting experts.

Could the Rifle Have Done It?

The Commission had various tests made purportedly to evaluate the accuracy of the weapon said to have been used in the murder. The Commission Report summarized the results as follows.

Accuracy of Weapon

... the assassin in all probability hit two out of the three shots during the maximum time span of 4.8 to 5.6 seconds if the second shot missed, or, if either the first or third shots missed, the assassin fired the three shots during a minimum time span of 7.1 to 7.9 seconds. A series of tests were performed to determine whether the weapon and ammunition used in the assassination were capable of firing the shots which were fired by the assassin on November 22, 1963. The ammunition used by the assassin was manufactured by Western Cartridge Co. of East Alton, Ill. In tests with the Mannlicher-Carcano C2766 rifle, over 100 rounds of this ammunition were fired by the FBI and the Infantry Weapons Evaluation Branch of the U.S. Army. There were no misfires.

In an effort to test the rifle under conditions which simulated those which prevailed during the assassination, the Infantry Weapons Evaluation Branch of the Ballistics Research Laboratory had expert riflemen fire the assassination weapon from a tower at three silhouette targets at distances of 175, 240, and 265 feet. The target at 265 feet was placed to the right of the 240-foot target which was in turn placed to the right of the closest silhouette. Using the assassination rifle mounted with the telescopic sight, three marksmen, rated as master by the National Rifle Association, each fired two series of three shots. In the first series the firers required time spans of 4.6, 6.75, and 8.25 seconds respectively. On the second series they required 5.15, 6.45, and 7 seconds. None of the marksmen had any practice with the assassination weapon except for exercising the bolt for 2 or 3 minutes on a dry run. They had not even pulled the trigger because of concern about breaking the firing pin.

The marksmen took as much time as they wanted for the first target and all hit the target. For the first four attempts, the firers missed the second shot by several inches. The angle from the first to the second shot was greater than from the second to the third shot and required a movement in the basic firing position of the marksmen. This angle was used in the test because the majority of eyewitnesses to the assassination stated that there was a shorter interval between shots two and three than between shots one and two. As has been shown, if the three shots were fired within a period of from 4.8 to 5.6 seconds, the shots would have been evenly spaced and the assassin would not have incurred so sharp an angular movement.

Five of the six shots hit the third target where the angle of movement of the weapon was small. On the basis of these results, Simmons testified that in his opinion the probability of hitting the targets at the relatively short range at which they were hit was very high. Considering the various probabilities which may have prevailed during the actual assassination, the highest level of firing performance which would have been required of the assassin and the C2766 rifle would have been to fire three times and hit the target twice within a span of 4.8 to 5.6 seconds. In fact, one of the firers in the rapid fire test in firing his two series of three shots, hit the target twice within a span of 4.6 and 5.15 seconds. The others would have been able to reduce their times if they had been given the opportunity to become familiar with the movement of the bolt and the trigger pull. Simmons testified that familiarity with the bolt could be achieved in dry practice and, as has been indicated above, Oswald engaged in such practice. If the assassin missed either the first or third shot, he had a total of between 4.8 and 5.6 seconds between the two shots which hit and a total minimum time period of from 7.1 to 7.9 seconds for all three shots. All three of the firers in these tests were able to fire the rounds within the time period which would have been available to the assassin under those conditions.

Three FBI firearms experts tested the rifle in order to determine the speed with which it could be fired. The purpose of this experiment was not to test the rifle under conditions which prevailed at the time of the assassination but to determine the maximum speed at which it could be fired. The three FBI experts each fired three shots from the weapon at 15 yards in 6, 7, and 9 seconds, and one of these agents, Robert A. Frazier, fired two series of three shots at 25 yards in 4.6 and 4.8 seconds. At 15 yards each man's shots landed within the size of a dime. The shots fired by Frazier at the range of 25 yards landed within an area of 2 inches and 5 inches respectively. Frazier later fired four groups of three shots at a distance of 100 yards in 5.9, 6.2, 5.6, and 6.5 seconds. Each series of three shots landed within areas ranging in diameter from 3 to 5 inches. Although all of the shots were a few inches high and to the right of the target, this was because of a defect in the scope which was recognized by the FBI agents and which they could have compensated for if they were aiming to hit a bull's-eye. They were instead firing to determine how rapidly the weapon could be fired and the area within which three shots could be placed. Frazier said, "The fact that the crosshairs are set high would actually compensate for any lead which had to be taken. So that if you aimed with this weapon as it actually was received at the laboratory, it would not be necessary to take any lead whatsoever in order to hit the intended object. The scope would accomplish the lead for you." Frazier added that the scope would cause a slight miss to the right. It should be noted, however, that the President's car was curving slightly to the right when the third shot was fired.

Based on these tests the experts agreed that the assassination rifle was an accurate weapon. Simmons described it as "quite accurate," in fact, as accurate as current military rifles.* Frazier testified that the rifle was accurate, that it had

---

*Tests on the alleged murder rifle were reported in testimony by Simmons. A peculiar mathematical manipulation of the results took place and vitiated the test. First of all, the telescope sight system was rebuilt. The rifle was then fixed in a vise called a bench rest. The rifle was fired to discover its innate accuracy or lack of accuracy. After removal from the vise, the rifle was fired by three different experts at stationery targets. From the score of each shooter was subtracted the inherent lack of accuracy of the rifle. Simmons admitted they had subtracted out the round-to-round dispersion" (Hearings, vol. 3, pp. 294, 295, 241, 281-291). In other words, the test demonstrated the shooting abilities of three rifle experts who had nothing to do with the incident (a fact that was already known) firing a perfectly accurate rifle. It was a nontest and had absolutely no relevance to Oswald's ability to place shots in a moving target using the alleged murder weapon, which was so severely defective as to require significant gunsmithing before it could be "tested." (C.G.W.)

less recoil than the average military rifle and that one would not have to be an expert marksman to have accomplished the assassination with the weapon which was used.

Conclusion

The various tests showed that the Mannlicher-Carcano was an accurate rifle and that the use of a four-power scope was a substantial aid to rapid, accurate firing. Oswald's Marine training in marksmanship, his other rifle experience and his established familiarity with this particular weapon show that he possessed ample capability to commit the assassination. Based on the known facts of the assassination, the Marine marksmanship experts, Major Anderson and Sergeant Zahm, concurred in the opinion that Oswald had the capability to fire three shots, with two hits, within 4.8 and 5.6 seconds. Concerning the shots which struck the President in the back of the neck, Sergeant Zahm testified: "With the equipment he [Oswald] had and with his ability I consider it a very easy shot." Having fired this shot the assassin was then required to hit the target one more time within a space of from 4.8 to 5.6 seconds. On the basis of Oswald's training and the accuracy of the weapon as established by the tests, the Commission concluded that Oswald was capable of accomplishing this second hit even if there was an intervening shot which missed. The probability of hitting the President a second time would have been markedly increased if, in fact, he had missed either the first or third shots thereby leaving a time span of 4.8 to 5.6 seconds between the two shots which struck their mark. The Commission agrees with the testimony of Marine marksmanship expert Zahm that it was "an easy shot" to hit some part of the President's body, and that the range where the rifleman would be expected to hit would include the President's head.

An Evaluation of the Rifle

Askins (1969) maintains that the 6.5 millimeter Mannlicher-Carcano cartridge is a "good round." The case is 52 millimeters long, rimless, bottleneck; head diameter, 0.447 inch; rim, 0.446

inch; neck, 0.296 inch. Standard Italian World War II service rounds have a bullet that weighs 159 grains; muzzle velocity 2225 feet per second; average breech pressure, about 39,000 pounds per square inch.

War surplus models of this gun in the rifle or in the carbine version are usually of poor accuracy; bore dimensions are uncertain; head space is questionable. Trigger pull is impossibly bad in all guns of this model; extensive work by a skilled gunsmith is required before these guns can be shot with any semblance of accuracy.

Norma produces a cartridge for this gun that is 156 grains; soft-nosed, round-nosed bullet; muzzle velocity 2,000 feet per second.

The 6.5 millimeter brass for these cartridges is available; it is all Berdan-primed. The cartridge is effective; the rifle for it is at best mediocre. The evaluation of the rifle by the Warren Commission was clearly incompetent.

Be that as it may, it is not unreasonable to suggest that, if indeed the single rifle single assassin conclusion of the Commission were valid, then a most unusual outcome occurred. The combination of an intrinsically poor rifle in poor condition fired by an indifferent shooter resulted in a degree of accuracy on a moving target at a rapid fire rate that could not be equaled by some of the best riflemen available in the United States.

Bullet Fragments in Kennedy's Body

Mr. Frazier of the FBI testified that he received two metal fragments from agents of the Baltimore FBI office, "who stated that they had obtained these in the autopsy room of the Naval Hospital near Washington, D.C. where they were present when they were removed from the head of President Kennedy" (Commission Exhibit No. 843).

The fragments were lead; one piece weighed 1.65 grains, the other 0.15 grain. A spectrographic analysis was said to have been done. These particles from the President's head were compared to a fragment from Govenor Connally's arm, to lead scrapings from the inside of the windshield, and to three lead fragments found in on the rear floorboard carpet of the limousine, as well as to a bullet fragment found on the front seat of the automobile in which the President had been riding. "... they were found to be similar in metallic composition." Further, "... they are of similar lead composition."

The Frazier statement is of course meaningless since "similar in metallic composition" says nothing. A slug of type metal could be called "of similar lead composition" to a lead bullet fragment.

Only a study of the detailed spectrographic results would permit one to evaluate the conclusions expressed by Frazier.

Bullet Fragments in Kennedy's Head

Secret Service Agent Kellerman testified that he examined, with the pathologists, x-rays of the late President's head. His comments made under oath follow. "From the x-rays, when you placed the x-rays up against the light the whole head looked like a mass of stars, there must have been 30, 40 lights where these pieces were so minute that they couldn't be reached." Apparently the only piece of lead removed by the pathologists from the President's head region was a fragment "that was above the right eye."

This layman's description of the head x-rays made of the President's remains suggests an almost explosive fragmentation of the bullet that struck the head. Such breakup of a bullet is characteristic of soft-nosed hunting bullets; it is not characteristic of military bullets that have a lead core covered by a copper metal jacket. In fact, military bullets are by international custom so constructed as to obviate explosive wounds.

Despite this peculiar behavior of the bullet, government scientists assured Mr. Specter, attorney for the Commission, that it was quite to be expected and that a military bullet could so perform. At high velocities, massive wounds and fragmentation of the skull can occur along the suture lines. Such high-velocity bullets "may pulp the brain substance" (Wilber, 1974). Velocities which cause such explosive-type wounds with military-style bullets are usually 2000 feet per second or greater. At such velocities temporary pulsating cavities (often twenty-six times the volume of the permanent cavity produced by tunneling of the bullet) are formed and the process results in destruction of bone and tissue far removed from the actual bullet tunnel (Wilber, 1974).

The question arises whether the impact velocity of a Mannlicher-Carcano 6.5 mm bullet striking at the distance between shooter and Kennedy's head was 2000 feet per second or more.

The Bullet Velocities

The testimony of Doctor Olivier, a veterinarian who performed shooting tests with 6.5 mm Mannlicher-Carcano cartridges using goats and blocks of gelatin as targets, indicated that such bullets fired from about seventy yards distance into a goat and striking the rib were flattened at the nose end. Commission Exhibit Number 853 shows one of these test-fired bullets.

Olivier fired other 6.5 mm Mannlicher-Carcano cartridges at the wrists of human cadavers, producing comminuted fractures. The sample fired bullet in Commission Exhibit Number 856 shows that the nose was severely deformed and flattened as a result of striking wrist bone. Indeed the nose had a concave configuration.

A balance sheet of velocities and energies of the 158-grain Mannlicher-Carcano bullet as it passed through the various structures the Commission concluded it traversed according to their single bullet theory raises a number of questions. The following balance sheet was constructed from data sworn to by Edgewood Arsenal ballistic scientists in testimony before the Warren Commission. The data were obtained from tests using simulations of the President's body tissues, Connally's rib, and Connally's wrist. Recall that the cartridges alleged to have been used held bullets weighing about 158 grains. The following formula is used to calculate energies. The answer will be in foot pounds of energy.

$$E = mv^2/2g \ 7000 \text{ or } mv^2/450,000$$

Location of Bullet	Velocity in feet per second	Energy in foot pounds
Muzzle of rifle	2160	1638
At 60 yards	1900	1268
After passing through JFK body	1779	1111
After passing through simulated Connally rib	1514	805
After passing through Connally's wrist	1432	720

The residual velocity is that which was left in the bullet said to have entered Connally's thigh, striking the bone and leaving a piece of metal in the thigh bone. The bullet was then said to have backed out of the leg wound and fallen onto a stretcher.

One might argue that this table based on simulated targets has overestimated the residual velocities and energies. Assume that the estimate is cut in half. It then is apparent that the bullet entering Connally's leg (in accord with the Commission theory) had a velocity of at least 716 feet per second and a striking energy of 360 foot pounds. These values are similar to those encountered when an Army .45 automatic pistol is fired at near-contact range. Since energy is the key factor in wound production, the following table of comparison should be used in evaluating the energy relations that seem to be part of the single bullet theory.

Bullet in question	Energy in foot pounds
Pristine bullet entering Connally's thigh	360
.45 Army Auto., muzzle	369
.38 Special, muzzle	265
9 mm Luger, muzzle	345
.44 Special, muzzle	295
.22 Winchester Magnum, muzzle	356

If the Edgewood Arsenal data are correct and the Commission one bullet theory is valid, the bullet striking Connally in the thigh should have produced results much like a pistol shot at near-contact range made with one of the rounds listed above.

Olivier testified that "the bullet that passed through the President's neck had lost very little of its wounding potential and was capable of doing a great deal of damage in penetrating." As one example of the "terrific" penetrating capacity of the bullet, it was reported to have gone through 72.5 centimeters (about 28 inches) of 20% gelatin and then buried itself in a mound of earth (Hearings, vol. V, p. 78).

Later, under circuitous questioning by attorney Specter, Olivier seems to change his emphasis on how terrific the power of the bullet was; he seems to attempt to show how little energy was left to damage Connally's wrist and thigh.

The lack of significant deformation of the bullet that allegedly inflicted the nonfatal wounds on Kennedy and on Connally was nowhere clarified in a meaningful way.

Olivier's later testimony to the effect that the bullet that struck Connally's thigh was "spent" and thus just entered the leg after which it fell out onto a stretcher does not account for the metal fragment left in the thigh bone, nor the energy needed to perforate the skin and penetrate muscle to the bone. Had the bullet penetrated the leg to the bone under low velocity, why did not the muscle tissues and the thigh skin contract to hold the missile in place?

Doctor George T. Shires, who was Professor of Surgery and Chairman of the Department at Southwestern Medical School, treated the gunshot wound in the thigh of the Governor. Doctor Shires had been certified by the American Board of Surgery in 1956. According to his report, "there was a 1 cm. [about 0.4 of an inch] punctate missile wound over the juncture of the middle and lower third, medical aspect of the left thigh. X-rays of the thigh and leg revealed a bullet fragment which was imbedded in the body of the femur in the distal third" *Texas Journal of Medicine,* 1964).

Doctor Shires explored the wound after the usual surgical preparation of the area. "The missile wound was seen to course through the subcutaneous fat and into the vastus medialis. The necrotic fat and muscle were debrided [cut away] down to the region of the femur. The direction of the missile wound was judged not to be in the course of the femoral vessel, since the wound was distal and anterior to Hunter's canal" (*Texas Journal of Medicine,* 1964).

The punctate wound suggested a bullet entering the leg nose downward and not wobbling particularly. The 1 cm diameter is about 0.4 inch; the 6.5 mm bullet has a caliber of about 0.26 inch.

Cartridge Quality

The question of quality of the ammunition used in the alleged murder rifle was suggested by information available from the manufacturers.

In a letter dated 14 July 1965 H.J. Gebelein, Assistant Sales Service Manager, Winchester-Western Division of Olin Mathieson Corporation, stated that at the time of his letter the 6.5 millimeter Mannlicher-Carcano cartridge was not being produced commercially. He further stated that any former production of the cartridge had been under government contracts, all of which were terminated upon completion of the work in 1944. He concluded that ". . . any of this ammunition which is on the market today is Government surplus ammunition" (Gebelein, 1965).

It is obvious that the ammunition used in the assassination was either war surplus cartridges nearly twenty years old at the time of firing or reloaded (handloaded) cartridges. In the former case the vaunted reliability and top quality of the ammunition might be properly questioned. If some of the cartridges were handloads, hunting-style bullets in all probability were used rather than military-style, full metal-jacket bullets.

There is some information to the effect that reloaded 6.5 mm Mannlicher-Carcano ammunition was available commercially in the United States.

The Bullets

A critical difficulty confronts the scholar who attempts to

clarify the issue of what bullets were fired, from what point, and where the bullets came to rest.

According to the Commission, a single undeformed bullet (other than for rifling marks and a lateral compression of the base) was found in Parkland Hospital. The Commission contended that the undeformed bullet had passed through the bodies of Kennedy and Connally, smashing two bones in the latter's body and leaving a piece of metal in the Governor's thigh bone.

No other whole bullet was found. The bullet hole in the limousine windshield was unresolved. There was evidence of a shot that came from behind the limousine and struck the windshield. The so-called Altgen's photograph showed the resulting hole. A reporter, Richard Dudman, referred to the bullet hole. Sergeant Stavis Ellis reportedly described the hole in the windshield as large enough to admit a pencil. The spent 6.5 mm cartridge cases found in the Book Depository Building were said by the Commission to have been chambered in the alleged assassination rifle. There was some question in the mind of observers about one of the cartridges, which may have been deformed in such a manner as to have precluded its holding a bullet in the neck. Vigorous ejection of a spent case often results in distortion at the neck.

The Commission claimed that such cartridges were readily available to sportsmen, a claim open to serious doubt.

Apparently no examination was made to ascertain whether these cases had been reloaded by hand. By implication at least, the cartridges used by the assassin were surplus 6.5 mm military-style rounds.

The fatal head wound to the President was explosive in nature. So extensive was the damage to the skull that the brain almost fell out by gravity; virtually no work with the autopsy saw was needed to break the brain loose. Clearly identifiable pieces of metal were scattered about the head and brain of the deceased according to recently released x-rays of the shattered head (Wilber, 1977). A sizeable piece of metal was shown at the entrance wound, a fact strongly indicative of a lead-nosed bullet. No intact or deformed bullet that caused the head wound was clearly reported in the official documents of the Commission.

According to the Commission, the spent cartridges used in the murder were all found. One pristine bullet said to have been used in the attempt was found. The only shots fired were said to have been those through the alleged murder rifle using the few cartridges on record. No other cartridges of that type were found anywhere and certainly not in any of Oswald's possessions. It is not usual to purchase one or two rifle cartridges. Ordinarily a box of twenty or box of fifty is the smallest unit of sale. Where are the remainder of the cartridges that Oswald would have had to purchase?

If all the cartridges used were the reliable quality that the Commission emphasized, as is usual with fresh commercial ammunition, the variability in performance from one to another would have been negligible, especially if fired through the same rifle in a brief moment of time.

Accepting that all the bullets were from essentially identical high quality cartridges fired by an expert from the same rifle from the same position in all instances, it is difficult to understand how one of the bullets fired under these conditions disintegrated explosively as it passed through the single layer of flat bone of the President's skull, whereas another virtually identical cartridge under identical conditions drove its bullet into a rib, smashing it, through a wrist bone of a large man, causing a comminuted fracture, left metal en route in Connally's body, including a piece still in this thigh, and yet remained in an undeformed and undamaged condition except for the rifling engraved on the sides. The disparity of deformation of the bullets between what happened to the head wound bullet and what was said to have happened to the nonlethal wound bullet was so great as to raise doubts, from a ballistic point of view, that the bullet that struck the President's head was of the same construction as the pristine bullet that inflicted the nonlethal injuries to two men.

The President's head wound was so massive as to suggest its production by a hunting-style bullet, despite the attempts at disclaimer by Doctor Humes led on by lawyer Specter. A semi-jacketed bullet with a soft lead nose exposed would be more likely to produce the kind of head wound described at autopsy of the President than would a metal-jacketed military bullet similar to the undeformed slug that was presented as having been found on a stretcher in Parkland Hospital.

The bullet fragments later found in the presidential limousine were reported to have come from the rifle owned by Oswald. Obviously at least one bullet fragmented; an allegedly similar bullet (the pristine one) did not, although it impacted heavier bone than did the fragmented one.

Were there bits of bone and tissue on the bullet fragments found in the limousine? Could that material have been blood-typed and otherwise subjected to biological analysis?

Bullet Fragments in Connally

Were the bullet fragments removed from Connally's body identical in chemical constitution to the mysterious bullet (Commission Exhibit No. 399) that was found in Parkland Memorial Hospital?

A secret letter to the Commission from J. Edgar Hoover on 8 July 1964 admitted that a spectrographic analysis of the bullet pieces taken from Connally's body gave no useful information (Wecht, 1974).

The fragments from Connally's body and Commission Exhibit Number 399 were compared using neutron activation analysis. Hoover also conceded in his letter that "minor variations" were recorded between Commission Exhibit Number 399 and the pieces of metal taken from Connally's body by his surgeons.

In 1975 the supposedly complete report of the activation analysis was released. It consisted of raw data of the first order, i.e. it was essentially bench-level laboratory notes. To date, examination of the FBI "report" on the activation analysis showed in truth that it was not adequate.

Modern sophisticated neutron activation analysis might give an answer. But at present, there are no data to indicate that the bullet fragments taken from Connally's body are or are not identical in composition to Commission Exhibit Number 399.

Identification of Bullet Fragments

It has been suggested that analysis of the various fragments of bullets found in the Kennedy assassination case might result in the pinpointing of just where the fragments came from. Were they all from similar bullets? Where they all from war surplus Mannlicher-Carcano ammunition?

The FBI was said to have taken various samples of the fragments found as well as a small piece of the undeformed bullet found at Parkland Hospital; later these samples were subjected to trace metal analysis. No clear-cut results have been made public. At the time the analytical work was done, the technology of such chemical analysis was not sufficiently advanced to permit precise characterization of bullets in this manner.

It is now possible to clearly distinguish similar ammunition made by different manufacturers one from another (Guy and Pate, 1973). The precise characterization of a given bullet is still not feasible. Tests run on the copper jackets of bullets that have them are more clean-cut and show great promise with respect to bullet characterization (Guy and Pate, 1973). The bullets themselves (the lead slugs) have an overwhelming antimony radioactivity after radiation by the neutron source. Hence even minute amounts of antimony in the lead bullet cause interference with the results.

At the present time neutron activation analysis of bullets for the purpose of characterization shows early promise, but the state of the art is not such that the method and results could be used in court. It is doubtful that significant information can come from the analytical work done on the Kennedy-Connally bullets and fragments.

Organic Matter on Bullets

A serious oversight from the crime investigation point of view was the lack of any apparent attempt by the FBI or other agency to identify blood or other tissue on the single bullet said to have caused the nonfatal wounds to the President and to Connally or on bullet fragments collected. Sophisticated crime investigators such as the FBI agents are said to be should have been aware of the value of blood and tissue on a spent bullet which went through a victim or two.

Foreign material on such a bullet or fragment might include blood, muscle, fibers, or bone. Blood could be typed; tissues could be identified as being human or not. Fibers, if found, could be compared with the cloth of garments through which the bullet was said to have passed. Skilled biomedical laboratory technicians could have typed any blood on the bullet and compared the result with the known blood types of Kennedy and Connally. Why was such an investigation not carried out?

It cannot be argued that such tests are unusual or esoteric. They are part of any routine competent medicolegal investigation of a gunshot wound case.

Were such tests made on the bullet fragments found on the floor of the presidential limousine? The record does not say. Again, if the fragments were not tested for foreign materials, e.g. brain tissue, blood, why were they not?

The Shots Fired

To what conclusions does the complex of evidence lead with respect to the number of shots and where they went?

The angles above the horizontal of two of the shots are such as to demand fairly firm conclusions. The angle of the shot that caused the nonfatal wounds in Connally was about 25 degrees downward from the horizontal. The shot that caused the nonfatal wound in Kennedy was along the horizontal or slightly upward. The lateral orientation of the two nonfatal wounds was such as to indicate that two separate and distinct bullets, coming from different points of origin but both probably from behind the two men, were involved (Wilber, 1977).

The Federal Bureau of Investigation asserts the following in a voluminous but not commendable report. "As the motorcade was traveling through downtown Dallas on Elm Street about fifty yards west of the intersection with Houston Street . . . three shots rang out. Two bullets struck President Kennedy, and one wounded Governor Connally. The President, who slumped forward in the car, was rushed to Parkland Memorial Hospital, where he was pronounced dead at 1:00 p.m."

This digest of the shooting is in accord with the observations of seasoned newsmen who filed stories during those early hours after the murder. It is in accord with the testimony of numerous police officers who were in the vicinity. It is in accord with the testimony of Governor Connally and his wife.

The FBI summary report further admitted that "immediately after President Kennedy and Governor Connally were admitted to Parkland Memorial Hospital, a bullet was found on one of the stretchers. Medical examination of the President's body revealed that one of the bullets had entered just below his shoulder to the right of the spinal column at an angle of 45 to 60 degrees downward, that there was no point of exit, and that the bullet was not in the body. An examination of this bullet by the FBI Laboratory determined that it had been fired from the rifle owned by Oswald."

The problem of the angle of the shot described has never been satisfactorily resolved. It probably resulted from a misunderstanding of conversation by the pathologists during the time that they were conducting their examination.

What seems clear is that one bullet struck Kennedy and inflicted a nonfatal wound. Another bullet struck Connally and inflicted a number of serious wounds that proved to be nonfatal. A third shot was fatal for Kennedy.

The Commission's theory that a single bullet caused the nonfatal wounds in both Kennedy and Connally cannot be squared with the available data nor with the basic laws of ballistics. For example, rifle bullets, although they may do strange things and take odd paths through living flesh, do not perform such bizarre actions as to make one or more right-angle turns in midair. Nor do bullets, even fully metal-jacketed ones, driven at fairly high velocities strike bone without showing measurable signs of deformation.

It is questionable that the mysterious bullet referred to in the FBI report and used by the Commission as the key exhibit in its one bullet theory ever passed through either Kennedy or Connally. If it had, there would have been traces of blood, tissue, body fluid, and even thread from clothing. In all probability there would have been sufficient biological material stuck to the bullet to permit the identification of blood type. In view of the fact that no such findings were reported anywhere in the Report or Hearings, it is safe to conclude that the pristine bullet never passed through human flesh.

All the pathologists and the surgeons who attended Governor Connally agreed that the so-called pristine bullet found on a stretcher could not have caused the extensive injuries to Connally; there just was not enough metal missing from the mysterious slug to balance what was found in the Governor.

The massive head wound of the President should be clearcut, but the strange behavior of the Commission concerning all the autopsy findings and the subsequent outrageous secrecy game played by federal custodians of the Commission fi'es have muddied matters so badly as to throw into doubt almosι all the Commission has reported.

It seems that there was a single shot from behind that entered the President's head somewhere between the top of his skull and the occipital region just to the right of the midline. Massive destruction of the brain and skull resulted. A flap of skin or scalp on the back of the head has never been adequately described. Could it have been an exit wound of a bullet fragment or piece of bone? A strange foreign object of some sort, seen in one of the photographs of the brain, has never been adequately evaluated.

From the ballistic point of view the extent of destruction of the President's brain and skull suggests that perhaps a military-style bullet was not used for that shot. The massive wound is more characteristic of the wounds seen after shooting with a soft-nosed hunting-style bullet.

The so-called evidence of a shot to the head from in front of the President based on motion picture analysis is nonpersuasive. It is based on misunderstanding of the laws of momentum. A disturbing report from Parkland Hospital to the effect that there was a wound to the left temple was never adequately evaluated by the Commission nor anyone else who probed the case. It is now too late in all probability to clarify that issue. Massive destruction to the right side of the head is compatible with an entry wound to left temporal region.

The Warren Commission came to a conclusion about the Kennedy murder based on evaluation of the rifle, cartridges, and the suspect's abilities and behavior. The Commission contended that "on the basis of evidence . . . the Commission has found that Lee Harvey Oswald (1) owned and possessed the rifle used to kill President Kennedy and wound Governor Connally, (2) brought this rifle into the Depository Building on the morning of the assassination, (3) was present, at the time of the assassination, at the window from which the shots were fired, (4) killed Dallas Police Officer J.D. Tippit in an apparent attempt to escape, (5) resisted arrest by drawing a fully loaded pistol and attempting to shoot another police officer, (6) lied to the police after his arrest concerning important substantive matters, (7) attempted, in April 1963, to kill Maj. Gen. Edwin A. Walker, and (8) possessed the capability with a rifle which would have enabled him to commit the assassination. On the basis of these findings the Commission has concluded that Lee Harvey Oswald was the assassin of President Kennedy."

The problem of the rifle and its accuracy remains. How the suspect Oswald could have performed so outstandingly as a shooter on that day in Dallas is still difficult to understand. Most of the confusion, contradictions, and questions surrounding the alleged murder weapon, the cartridges, and the lone suspect may never be resolved.

One matter does seem clear from an examination of the rifle and cartridge material. It is extremely doubtful that one shooter could have carried out the rapid, accurate firing at a moving target with the weapon said to have been used. At least two riflemen seem more probable.

CHAPTER 8

CRITIQUE:
THE NONFATAL WOUNDS

The Anterior Throat Wound

THE doctors at Parkland Hospital who observed the anterior throat wound and were able to come to a conclusion referred to it as punctate, round in outline, and having the general appearance of an entrance wound (an in-shoot). It was only a few millimeters in diameter. These observations were confirmed by the head nurse in the emergency room, a woman with extensive experience in the identification and treatment of bullet wounds.

According to further information, Doctor Perry "extended" the wound a few millimeters on either side in order to insert a tracheotomy tube in place. (In passing, it is of interest that Kennedy's personal physician, Admiral Burkley, made no reference to the anterior throat wound in the document signed by him and published as an official death certificate; the back wound was recognized and located anatomically in the document.)

When the President's remains were studied at autopsy, the anterior throat wound was discovered to be nearly 3 inches in length and was said to have gaping irregular edges.

A scientific conference, on a face-to-face basis, of all the doctors involved in the emergency procedures carried out at Parkland Memorial Hospital plus the three autopsy pathologists all having immediate access to the photographs and x-rays could have resulted in a valid and meaningful interpretation of the anterior throat wound. In view of the overwhelming importance of the case, failure to insure such a conference is unexplainable on the basis of oversight or ignorance.

Federal investigative agency officials, working within the

system that they are wedded to, are just not that absent-minded, uninformed, or readily demoralized to permit the excuse that such a routine and sane conference was not thought of in the confusion of the times.

A medicolegal conference, unsullied by the presence of non-medical personnel or medical personnel who were not operatively involved in the case on a firsthand basis could have satisfactorily resolved the other strange aspects of the murder of President Kennedy. Neglect of such consultation defies explanation.

Failure to dissect the postulated bullet track between back and anterior throat was contrary to accepted standards of practice in forensic pathology.

The wound in the back of the President was not fatal. Its precise location has been confused by the careless and apparently planned misuse of terms in locating this wound. According to Commander Humes' testimony, this wound in the back "was situated just above the upper border of the scapula, and measured 7 x 4 millimeters, with its long axis roughly parallel to the long axis of the vertical [*sic*] column." Presumably "vertebral column" is meant, or is it? (Hearings, vol. 2, p. 361) (*see* Fig. 8-3).

It might be appropriate to comment on the general attitude of apprehensiveness shown by Doctor Hume and his servility to Mr. Specter, lawyer for the Commission, and to the Commission as a whole. His discomfort suggests that he was under severe stress of some sort. Colonel Pierre Finck's nervous behavior during his testimony and his behavior afterwards suggests that he felt threatened in some way. What kind of threats or retributions were held over the heads of these medical men? The internal evidence of their testimonies suggests something of this sort was, in fact, causing them to be ill-at-ease far beyond what one would anticipate as a result of these formal hearings.

According to the Report (p. 89), the anterior throat wound in the President's remains was small and round in outline. "Dr. Charles S. Carrico, a resident surgeon at Parkland, noted a small wound approximately one-fourth of an inch in diameter (5 to 8 millimeters) in the lower third of the neck below the Adam's apple. Dr. Malcolm O. Perry, who performed the tracheotomy, described the wound as approximately one-fifth of an inch in diameter (5 millimeters) and exuding blood which partially hid edges that were 'neither cleancut, that is, punched out, nor were they very ragged.'" Later questioning of these doctors by staff lawyers skillfully using the "hypothetical question" technique merely confused the issue and twisted what the direct observations at the emergency room obviously were.

Doctor Carrico, in his signed admission note, explained that a special tube was inserted down the President's throat into his windpipe to assist his breathing. During the manipulation "through the laryngoscope a ragged wound of the trachea was seen immediately below the larynx. The tube was passed past the laceration and the cuff inflated."

Later, according to Doctor Robert N. McClelland, "Drs. Perry, Baxter and I then performed a tracheotomy for respiratory distress and tracheal injury and Drs. Jones and Paul Peters inserted bilateral anterior chest tubes for pneumothoracis secondary to tracheomediastinal injury" (Report, p. 526).

It is apparent that the injury to the right side of the trachea was ragged and larger than the small hole in the anterior throat skin. Under ordinary circumstances it would be concluded that the small round hole in the skin was an entrance hole and that the larger tear in the trachea resulted from bullet wobble caused by passage of the missile through the skin and then partially into the trachea. This observation is not original with this author; it was originally aired by Doctor Nathan Jones in a letter to the editor of *Ramparts* (1967).

With respect to the wound in the lower neck, the upper back, or the back of the President, it is not clear which term is being used precisely, on page 361 of the Hearings, volume 2, the wound is located 14 cm from the tip of the mastoid process and 14 cm from the acromion; the right acromion process was specified. An interesting point was made by Doctor Humes; he said that "attempts to probe the vicinity of this wound were unsuccessful without fear of making a false passage." When asked to explain this statement he said, "I thought that it was impossible to take probes [metal rods which are used to poke into wounds so that one can find the pathway through tissue] and arrive at a definite pathway of the bullet beyond the surface of the muscles." The defect in the front part of the neck was described as a recent surgical defect in the lower anterior neck which measured some 7 or 8 cm in length. The location is rather vague concerning the head of the breastbone or some such structure as that.

The firsthand report of Doctor Humes' discovery of the back wound in the President's remains is informative. A hole that looked like a bullet hole was found "below the shoulders" and "two inches to the right of the middle line of the spinal column."

The report from the FBI went on, "this opening was probed by Dr. Humes with the finger, at which time it was determined that the trajectory of the missile entering at this point had entered at a downward position of 45 to 60 degrees. Further probing determined that the distance travelled by this missile was a short distance inasmuch as the end of the opening could be felt with the finger."

The confusion over this hole with no bullet in the corpse according to the x-rays was alleviated when information was given to Doctor Humes by FBI Special Agent Killion that a spent 6.5 mm rifle bullet was found on a stretcher at the hospital in Dallas. Humes then concluded that probably the bullet had struck the President in the back and caused a shallow wound. Later in the emergency room of the hospital the vigorous rescusitative endeavors of the surgeons worked loose the bullet which fell out somewhere. Its history from the emergency room to the stretcher in another area is not known (*see* Fig. 8-1, p. 195).

The author suggests that in cleaning up the emergency room after Kennedy's corpse was removed, some worker picked up the bullet. Later, after observing the savage, undisciplined behavior of Secret Service agents in and around the hospital (one even brutalized an FBI agent who happened to walk near him), the worker prudently dumped the bullet at a convenient "place of opportunity" in order to avoid an unpleasant situation.

As an aid in locating wounds in the body of any gunshot victim, clothing is an important item. The clothing of the murdered President was apparently seen by the doctors who did the autopsy only the day before Doctor Humes actually made his testimony. He said on page 364 of the Hearings, volume 2, "Yesterday, just shortly before the Commission hearing today was begun, Mr. Chief Justice, we had opportunity for the first time to examine the clothing worn by the late President." It is rather strange for the pathologists to first have access to the clothing in order to clarify the exact location of a wound months after the autopsy.

Mr. Specter, the lawyer, asked Doctor Humes, "Would it be accurate to state that the hole which you have identified as being the point of entry is approximately 6 inches below the top of the collar, and 2 inches to the right of the middle seam of the coat?" Commander Humes said, "That is approximately, sir. The defect, I might say, continues on through the material." Therefore, it seems clear that the nonfatal wound in what has been called a number of times the lower neck of the President was located with reference to the suit coat he wore 6 inches below the top of the collar and 2 inches to the right of the middle back seam. On an average man that would bring the bullet wound at the medial border of the right scapula and about one third of the way down from the top of the scapula.

Doctor Humes was also shown the blood-stained shirt worn by the President on the day he was murdered. He identified a hole in the back of the shirt and then two holes, one on either side of the neck fly of the shirt, in the front.

Mr. Specter asked Doctor Humes, "Would it be accurate to state that the hole in the back of the shirt is approximately 6 inches below the top of the collar and 2 inches to the right of the middle seam of the shirt?" Doctor Humes answered, "That is approximately correct, sir." When one looks at the Commission Exhibit Number 394 on page 25 of volume 17, it is difficult to know whether there is a central seam down the back of the President's shirt. The bullet hole in the back of the shirt is circled so that the reader can see it clearly. The shirt seems to be folded in a way which suggests a central seam going down the back. Ordinarily there is no seam down the middle of a man's shirt; seams usually run down the sides of a shirt and the back is made up of one entire piece of cloth. Perhaps the President's shirt was tailored a little differently than most shirts.

The point to be emphasized in this case, however, is that the holes of entry in both the coat and the shirt were admitted to be about 6 inches below the top of the collar in each garment.

Later, on page 366 of the Hearings, volume 17, Mr. McCloy, a member of the Commission, asked Doctor Humes, "Did your examination of the shirt, I just want to get it on the record, from your examination of the shirt, there is no defect in the collar of the shirt which coincides with the defect in the back of the President's coat, am I correct?" Doctor Humes answered without equivocation, "You are correct, sir. There is no such defect."

Thus, Humes' testimony emphasized that the hole in the back of Kennedy's suit coat was superimposable on the hole in his shirt.

Some Wound Evaluations

The autopsy team that carried out the postmortem examination of President Kennedy at Bethesda Naval Medical Center did not appreciate the fact that the wound in the late President's anterior throat region was, in fact, a bullet hole which had been modified surgically by attending physicians at Parkland Memorial Hospital.

It seems evident, then, that these pathologists could not make a competent judgment concerning the nature of the original hole in the anterior throat. Moreover, it is obvious that the staff lawyers of the Warren Commission had no competence whatsoever in the matter of gunshot wound interpretation. Specter, one of the lawyers, formulated the final theory of the shooting of John F. Kennedy presented by the Commission.

The unique characteristics of the anterior throat wound must be examined in the light of the observations made by attending surgeons at Parkland Memorial Hospital. These doctors were the only ones who actually saw the unmodified wound as it had been produced in the late President. Other observations made by pathologists after the body had been modified have little weight. Speculations by lawyers are valueless. It, therefore, seems appropriate to reexamine some of the observations made by trained and skilled surgeons who attempted to give medical aid to the stricken President.

Doctor R.N. McClelland, Associate Professor of Surgery at the University of Texas Southwestern Medical School, was interrogated by Arlen Specter under oath at great length concerning his role in treating the late President. Doctor McClelland had over 200 gunshot wound cases as part of his past professional experience (Hearings, vol. 6, p. 31). He was in a position to see intimately the details of the various wounds suffered by the President. He said in response to interrogation by Specter, "I was standing at the end of the stretcher on which the President was lying, immediately at his head, for purposes of holding a tracheotom, or a retractory in the neckline" (Hearings, vol. 6, p. 32). The neck wound was less than 0.25 inch in diameter. Doctor Perry described it carefully to Doctor McClelland as they consulted with one another.

Doctor Perry said that it was "a very small injury, with clearcut, although somewhat irregular margins of less than 1/4 inch in diameter with minimal tissue damage surrounding it on the skin" (Hearings, vol. 6, pp. 32-33). Doctor McClelland states further, "I was in such a position that I could very closely examine the head wound, and I noted that the right posterior portion of the skull had been extremely blasted. It had been shattered, apparently, by the force of the shot so that the parietal bone was protruded up through the scalp and seemed to be fractured almost along its right posterior half, as well as some of the occipital bone being fractured in its lateral half, and this sprung open the bones that I mentioned in such a way that you could actually look down into the skull cavity itself and see that probably a third or so, at least, of the brain tissue, posterior cerebral tissue and some of the cerebellar tissue had been blasted out. There was a large amount of bleeding which was occurring mainly from the large venous channels in the skull which had been blasted open" (Hearings, vol. 6, p. 33).

He also was of the opinion that the trachea had been "blasted or torn open by the fragments of the bullet."

The damage to the trachea and surrounding tissues was described. "The damage consisted mainly of a large amount of contusions and hematoma formation in the tissue lateral to the right side of the trachea and the swelling and bleeding around the site was to such extent that the trachea was somewhat deviated to the left side, not a great deal, but to a degree at least that it required partial cutting of some of the muscles in order to get good enough exposure to put in the tracheotomy tube, but there was a good deal of soft tissue damage and damage to the trachea itself where apparently the missile had gone between the trachea on the right side and the strap muscles which were applied closely to it" (Hearings, vol. 6, p. 33).

Specter, one of the lawyers for the Commission, asked Doctor McClelland whether, in fact, he had made the report said to be signed by him as part of Commission Exhibit Number 392. McClelland's answer was affirmative. Specter then asked, "And are all facts set forth true and correct to the best of your knowledge, information and belief?" Under oath, Doctor McClelland answered in the affirmative.

The part of the report of interest in evaluating the medical evidence connected with the assassination is simple and unequivocal. "The cause of death was due to massive head and brain injury from a gunshot wound of the left temple" (Commission Exhibit No. 392, vol. 17, pp. 11-12). This conclusion as to cause of death made by a qualified surgeon, with hundreds of gunshot wounds in his experience, standing immediately at the late President's head, has never been challenged by competent medical experts. It has been ignored. The weight of this opinion is of significance.

Despite harassment by Specter, who early in the hearings seemed to have already made up his mind what had happened, McClelland reaffirmed his professional opinion of the anterior neck wound. "If I saw the wound in its state in which Dr. Perry described it to me, I would probably initially think this were an entrance wound" (Hearings, vol. 6, p. 37).

Doctor Jenkins, a skilled, experienced anesthesiologist who had during sixteen years of service seen numerous gunshot wounds each week, replied to questioning by Specter. "I thought there was a wound at the left temporal area, right in the hairline and right above the zygomatic process" (Hearings, vol. 11, p. 48). Later, after harassment by Specter, Doctor Jenkins agreed that he modified his views as a result of reading various news reports and as a result of statements made to him by Specter.

Doctor Jones, another trained surgeon, described the throat wound as "a small wound at the midline of the neck, just above the supersternal notch, and this was probably no greater than one-fourth of an inch in greatest diameter" (Hearings, vol. 11, p. 53). He further indicated that there were no powder marks around the wound and that "there appeared to be a very minimal amount of disruption of [*sic*] [or?] interruption of the surrounding skin." The edges of the wound were smooth (Hearings, vol. 11, p. 54).

In Doctor Jones' written report he expressed the professional opinion that the anterior throat wound was an entrance wound (Hearings, vol. 11, p. 55; Doctor Jones' Exhibit No. 1, dated 23 November 1963). He gave an informed reason for his opinion. "The hole was very small and relatively clean cut as you would see in a bullet that is entering rather than exiting from a patient. If this were an exit wound, you would think that it exited at a very low velocity to produce no more damage than this had done, and if this were a missile of high velocity, you would expect more the explosive type of exit wound, with more tissue destruction than this appeared on superficial examination" (Hearings, vol. 11, p. 55).

Specter asked whether the anterior neck wound was compatible with a low-velocity bullet exiting at that point. Jones agreed that if the velocity of the bullet were so low that it barely fell out through the hole he might be able to understand how a hole of that nature could be made by a bullet exiting through the skin. Jones also admitted, during interrogation by

Specter, that he had treated during his residency no less than 150 gunshot cases and probably more.

Specter then attempted to harrass Jones and to show him up as unqualified. It was not an effective performance. Jones' testimony was clear, based on firsthand observation, and was compelling evidence of the anterior neck wound's being an entrance hole.

Doctor Kemp Clark was an agreeable witness for Arlen Specter. He was Head of the Neurological Surgery at Parkland Memorial Hospital. He admitted to signing the Kennedy death certificate in a murder case without approval by the local coroner. His reasoning was odd. He denied that it was negligent for him to sign the death certificate without adequate post-mortem examination, e.g. the body was not even turned over to examine the back before the certificate was signed. Clark's justification for this action follows. "In order to move the President's body to Bethesda where the autopsy was to be performed, a death certificate had to be filled out in conformation with Texas State law to allow the body to be transported. This is the second part of the signing of the death certificate" (Hearings, vol. 11, p. 30).

How did Doctor Clark know at the moment of the President's demise that the body would be autopsied at Bethesda? Had this been planned all along? Who told him of these plans? Who directed him to sign the death certificate? Was it in conformance with Texas state law for anyone but the coroner or medical examiner to sign a death certificate for a murdered victim? Was it the usual procedure for Doctor Clark to sign death certificates without autopsy data for patients who were shot in the streets of Dallas, were brought into his emergency room, and then died there as a result of gunshot wounds? Was this performance an example of collusion for some motive not made clear? Qualified surgeons were of the opinion that the throat wound of President Kennedy was made by a bullet entering the skin at that point. Moreover, the one doctor who was at the head of the stretcher and who had observed the President's head wounds in great detail referred to a bullet wound of the left temple as being the cause of death.

The anesthesiologist who handled the case maintained that he had observed a wound in the left temple located just about where Doctor McClelland said that it was. He obtained his impression from actual feeling of the skull with his hands in that particular area.

Table 8-I

SUMMARY OF OPINIONS ON ANTERIOR NECK WOUND
BY PARKLAND MEMORIAL HOSPITAL MEDICAL EXPERTS

Witness	*Reference*	*Anterior Neck Wound*
Doctor Carrico	pp. 5-6	Entrance wound
Doctor Perry	p. 14	Uncertain; punctate, smooth
Doctor Clark	p. 22	No information
Doctor McClelland	pp. 33, 35	Probably entrance wound
Doctor Baxter	p. 42	Not jagged; probably entrance
Doctor Jenkins	pp. 48, 51	Exit
Doctor Jones	pp. 55, 56	Clean-cut; entrance
Doctor Akin	pp. 65, 67	Punctate; possible entrance
Doctor Peters	p. 71	"Wound of entry in the throat"
Nurse Henchliffe	p. 143	"Entrance bullet hole"

The weight of opinion of the only medical personnel who saw the unmodified anterior neck wound in President Kennedy is that the clean-cut, punctate hole was an entrance wound (Hearings, vol. 6).

One may not discount, ignore, or distort such "on-the-scene" observation. It is true that when individuals under oath are subject to harrassment, bullying, and implied threats, they may find it convenient or even necessary to modify what they know to be the true observations made at the time of the occurrence. It is also true that with the passage of time, the impressions of observers of a scene or an incident become vague and less reliable. Details are lost as time passes and general impressions of a rudimentary sort remain. If one observes the evidence presented months after the incident to a hostile attorney and compares it with the evidence written out on the very day of the assassination by responsible, trained surgeons, there is no question that the latter reports must be given overwhelming weight in the face of later statements made under duress.

Triangulation

There is a perplexing aspect of the wound in the anterior throat of the late President as it was related to the wound in the back of the President. The Warren Commission came to the conclusion that the back wound was an entrance hole and that the anterior throat wound was the exit hole of the bullet that went in the back.

If the point of entrance of the nonfatal shot into the President's back is accepted according to Admiral Burkley's death certificate (at the level of the third thoracic vertebra), it would be possible to draw a line representing the bullet path horizontal to the ground or at right angles to the backbone at the level of the third thoracic vertebra. Such a line would go through the sternum as it exits the body just below the jugular notch. If the bullet were moving slightly from right to left as it perforated the body, it might strike the articular disc area at the sternoclavicular joint.

The location of the President in the limousine immediately before the shot makes such a path difficult to envision; the rear of the limousine might have served as a shield for such a theoretical shot.

If the angle of the line is rotated so that the bullet path is from behind at a downward angle of 10 degrees into the body, the path would lead into the sternum at the level of the second sternocostal joint. If the downward angle were 20 degrees, the bullet would have impacted at about the level of the third sternocostal joint.

The probable impaction sites are well below the injury reported in the President's anterior throat, where the wound was just below the larynx (the Adam's apple). In this region of the chest are the arch of the aorta and some of the large blood vessels of the body.

If an attempt is made to line up the back wound, as sworn to in the death certificate, with the anterior throat wound, avoiding all bony structures en route, the resulting path is somewhere between 10 and 15 degrees upward from the horizontal. Such an angle might have been created by a shooter firing from behind and slightly to the right of the limousine while standing or kneeling on the ground.

It is obvious that the nonfatal wound in Kennedy as described by the Warren Commission demanded a shooter at ground level and effectively precluded the causative bullet as coming from the sixth floor of the Texas Book Depository.

An alternative is that the back wound and the anterior throat wounds were unrelated. What happened to the bullet entering the President's back is unclear. What then caused the anterior throat wound? One suggestion has been that a bone fragment from the massive head wound exited the anterior throat (Thompson, 1976).

Moreover, the surgeons and the anesthesiologist at Parkland Memorial Hospital were under the impression that a bullet or bullet fragments had invaded the chest cavity of the late President. They based this conclusion on foam, froth, and blood that suggested to them that a pneumothorax had been created. A pneumothorax is a hole created in the chest cavity so that air leaks into the cavity; when it mixes with blood and body fluid, a foam results. The signs of a pneumothorax are well known to surgeons who function regularly in an emergency room. Because of this professional conclusion, the surgeons then proceeded to insert into the President's chest special tubes for reducing that pneumothorax and getting rid of the air so that the lungs of the stricken President could inflate and deflate naturally.

It is therefore perplexing that the autopsy pathologists found no evidence of the chest tubes actually having been inserted into the chest cavity. In addition, it is perplexing that no indication, according to the official report, of invasion of the chest cavity was seen at autopsy. If adequate photographs were taken during autopsy, the pictures of the chest cavity would have been helpful in evaluating this situation. Unfortunately, such photographs are not available, either through negligence at the time of autopsy, loss of the photographs subsequently, or official intransigence in keeping them secret.

Location of the Tracheal Wound

Where is the larynx located in the human body? "The larynx forms the anterior wall of the laryngeal part of the pharynx which separates it from the fourth, fifth and sixth cervical vertebrae" (Lockhart et al., 1972).

Below the larynx is the trachea, which begins at the level of the sixth cervical vertebra and extends downward for about 4 inches. Bifurcation into right and left bronchi respectively occurs at the level of the upper rim of the fifth thoracic vertebra and the sternal angle, about 2 inches below the jugular notch of the manubrium. The anterior wound of the President was in the cervical area of the trachea, at the level of about the third tracheal ring. Thus, it was located anatomically above the back wound, more toward the top of the head than was the back wound.

Photographs of the late President taken a moment before the shooting show him to be sitting in an upright position supported by a canvas and metal brace, which he found necessary to wear because his severe back injury caused him almost constant pain. Photographs taken at that time show no indication that the President was leaning forward or hunched over in a way that would raise the third thoracic vertebra to a level on the horizontal with the second and third tracheal ring. If the contention is accepted from the Burkley death certificate that the bullet that caused the nonfatal wounds in President Kennedy and Governor Connally entered the back of Kennedy at the level of the third thoracic vertebra, moved forward missing all hard structures and sliding between the muscle masses, and came out the anterior throat region, the bullet then took an upward course through the body.

At best, one is faced with an unresolved and perhaps unresolvable conflict between the observations of highly skilled and competent surgeons who saw an entrance wound in the anterior throat of the stricken President and nonscientific and technically incompetent individuals who say that the bullet entered the back and came out the throat, but in a downward direction.

The later behavior of that bullet is out of keeping with the facts as they are available. This nonfatal bullet is said to have left the anterior throat region of the President and is then said to have taken a downward course of 25 degrees from the horizontal. In addition, it made a right-angle turn to the right and another right-angle turn to the left so that it could enter the extreme right chest area of Governor Connally.

There is no way that this kind of bullet behavior can be supported by evidence. One must then look elsewhere for explanations of the severe wounds inflicted on Governor Connally. It has also been suggested that somehow or other the total body x-rays of the deceased President were inadequately done or inadequately interpreted. It seems probable that some bullet, bullets, or bullet fragments are still in the President's body.

Perhaps examination of the complete file of x-rays would clarify this point. Perhaps such a file of x-rays does not, in fact, exist. If the latter is true, there is no way to settle these serious discrepancies.

What can be seen, however, is the impossible conclusion presented by the Warren Commission. This conclusion is not in keeping with the facts presented to the Commission at its Hearings by responsible medical men. Apparently, the conclusion was the creation of one or more lawyers on the staff of the Commission. Why they felt that this end result fabricated out of whole cloth was necessary is obscure; it is not part of the subject of this presentation. However, these facts do suggest that others more competent to deal with social, political, and criminological matters should involve themselves in trying to find out why these very strange conclusions were, in fact, generated.*

---

*It must be emphasized that the autopsy pathologists at no time traced the path of the nonfatal wound through Kennedy's body. They never knew about the tracheotomy cut until the body had passed from their hands. Original notes and papers were burned; no firsthand tracing of the wound track was made. Observations by pathologist Doctor Finck and FBI observers indicated that the back wound was only about 2 inches deep and tunneled into the back at a downward angle of 45 to 60 degrees. It is thus clear that the "official" conclusions as to the back wound and the anterior neck wound are sheer speculation.

Time Sequence of the Rifle Shots

There seems to be little confusion or controversy over the speed of the film passing through the camera used by Abraham Zapruder to take the famous pictures of the assassination.

The FBI laboratory found that the film fed through the camera at about 18.3 frames per second. The Bell and Howell Company, according to a news story in the *New York Times* 8 December 1966, confirmed that speed.

According to the Warren Commission Report, page 97, it required an interval of 2.3 seconds between one shot and the next when firing the alleged assassination rifle. "Tests of the assassin's rifle disclosed that at least 2.3 seconds were required between shots."

The difficulty with using the Zapruder film for calibrating the time sequences is that there is no calibration of that film against the actual events. The film starts at no known precise point that can be given a time value. Hence there is no possible intermediate time value or end time value.

It is therefore of utmost importance that the motion picture films be interpreted cautiously. If the films seem to contradict what reliable data concerning the wound show, the latter must prevail.

The testimony of Governor Connally and his wife has great probative value in establishing the time sequence of shots.

Time Sequence

Despite the disclaimer in the Report, the single bullet theory of how Connally was wounded is crucial to the Commission's conclusions. Certain facts that were clearly evident from the Hearings themselves create difficulties for the single bullet theory.

The first and nonfatal wound of the late President and Governor Connally's wounds occurred within 1.5 seconds of one another. The rifle that the Commission concluded had been used to do the deed could not be fired that fast even by experts under ideal conditions. Tests run at the Commission's request clearly demonstrated that even after the rifle's scope sight system was rebuilt by ordnance experts, no expert could fire the rifle fast enough to get off succeeding shots within 1.5 seconds of one another. To save the theory, the Commission chose to ignore the results of its own tests in its Report.

A single bullet had to have caused the nonfatal wounds in Kennedy and Connally respectively or two separate and distinct rifles and riflemen had to have been involved; two bullets were fired but by two different shooters.

Another fact stands in the way of the single bullet theory. The single bullet found and claimed in the Report to have caused the nonfatal wounds in the late President and the Governor was minimally deformed; essentially it showed engravings on the surface from rifling and little more.

The Commission's own tests carried out at Edgewood Arsenal indicated that such a bullet could not have done what was claimed and still have remained in "pristine" condition. The autopsy surgeons unanimously denied that the undeformed bullet could have done what was claimed for it. In the Report the scientific evidence was ignored in favor of an incompetent hypothesis espoused by one of the lawyers to the Commission — a man with no ballistic qualifications on record.

It might be useful to recapitulate what the single bullet was supposed to have done and yet showed no significant deformation at the end of its flight. It entered and passed through the upper right part of the President's trunk, a path which carried it through back skin and anterior neck skin and through cartilage in the windpipe; in a most unusual fashion, it managed to avoid all other structures en route through the President and to slide between muscles. It exited from the front of the President's neck (according to the Report) going toward the left. It then made a right turn in midair until it was level with the extreme right side of the Governor, who was sitting directly in front of the President. Here it made a left turn in midair and plunged into the extreme right side of the Governor's back; in the process it tore out a large portion of the Governor's right fifth rib, shattering it and driving secondary bone missiles into the Governor's right lung. It exited just below the Governor's right nipple. It then entered his right wrist, shattering it and producing a comminuted fracture, leaving lead particles in that area. The bullet then entered the Governor's left thigh, driving a piece of metal into the thigh bone where it still resides. The bullet was then said to have backed out of the thigh wound and fallen on a stretcher, where it was claimed to have been found later in the day of the shooting.

In going through Connally, the following sheets of skin were perforated: back, anterior chest, anterior arm, posterior arm, thigh. Add these to the two sheets of skin perforated in passing through the President and there was a total of seven sheets of human skin (in addition to bone and muscle) perforated by the bullet that was claimed to be virtually undeformed (Fig. 8-1).

Perforation of Human Skin

Wound ballistic experts are familiar with the fact that human skin is difficult to perforate. A bullet passing through it loses a significant amount of energy. For example, a bullet loses about 161 feet per second of velocity in perforating a single layer of human skin (Wilber, 1974). As a general rule skin is more resistant to the passage of bullets than are other tissues. "For a 150 grain bullet to penetrate skin, a velocity of approximately 125 to 150 feet per second was required corresponding to approximately 5 foot pounds of energy" (Wilber, 1974).

It is reasonable to assume on the basis of calculations made from conclusions of Doctor Olivier, the federal veterinarian who did wounding tests for the Commission, that as much as 720 foot pounds of residual energy was left in the "single bullet" after it passed through Connally's wrist; that amount of energy would have been available to drive the bullet into Connally's thigh. Such a quantity of impact energy is slightly greater than the muzzle energy produced by the average .357

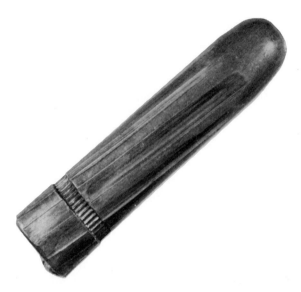

Figure 8-1. This is a photograph of Commission Exhibit Number 399, the mysterious bullet found after the murder of John F. Kennedy. The bullet is one from a 6.5 mm Mannlicher-Carcano cartridge; fully metal-jacketed except for the base, where the lead core is exposed. The rifling engraving on the sides of the bullet is clear. FBI studies established that this bullet was fired from the alleged murder rifle said to have been owned by Lee Harvey Oswald. The Commission concluded that this bullet had passed through Kennedy from back to front causing nonfatal wounds. It then supposedly passed through Connally, tearing out a portion of a rib on his right side, smashing his right wrist bone (comminuted fracture), and finally leaving a piece of metal in his left thigh. Note the undeformed state of the bullet.

Magnum revolver cartridge. The nature of Connally's thigh wound indicates a lesser residual energy for the bullet concerned as it moved into the deeper parts of the thigh (whether or not the "one bullet postulate" is accepted).

Seven sheets of human skin were perforated before the postulated single bullet entered Connally's thigh. Each sheet that was perforated absorbed 150 feet per second of velocity; the entire seven sheets then used up 1050 feet per second of the velocity of the perforating bullet. The residual velocity of the bullet as it drove into Connally's thigh muscle and bone was

850 feet per second, which is 1900 minus 1050 feet per second.

Taking the bullet weight at that time to be about 159 grains, the energy available to drive the bullet deep into the thigh was probably 255 foot pounds, a value roughly equivalent to the muzzle energy of a .38 Special revolver cartridge. In this argument no accounting has been made for the loss of velocity as a result of the bullet's smashing through Connally's rib bone and wrist bone.

The bone loss is partially balanced by the difference in presumed rifle to Kennedy range: The lawyer's hypothetical question gave 60 yards; the actual distance may have been more like 75 to 80 yards. The range of the later head shot was a little over 88 yards (Report, p. 110).

Bullet Deformation

Experimental study of the deformation of fully jacketed bullets striking bone indicates that velocity of impact plays a key role (Sellier, 1971). Passage through muscle per se leaves no markings on fully jacketed bullets.

When bullets that are fully jacketed with a metal covering (usually copper) strike bone, pronounced deformation results. Impact on skull bone at velocities of 1000 feet per second results in only a flattening of the nose of the bullet, but the deformation can be identified without equivocation.

If the bone struck is a long bone such as one in the arm or leg, the degree of deformation is much greater than follows upon striking of the skull plate. In all probability, the difference stems from the longer time of contact with the deforming force when the bullet strikes long bones as compared with the time when the bullet strikes the comparatively thin plate of the skull cap (Fig. 8-2).

If bone is covered with skin, e.g. the temporal bone, or with skin and muscle, e.g. the femur, the results are modified because skin and muscle absorb some of the impact energy before the bullet hits bone. For example, a bullet striking the head in the temporal region may have a velocity of 1000 feet per

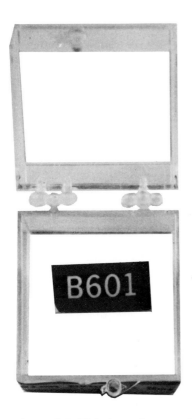

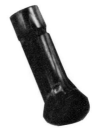

Figure 8-2. This is a photograph of Commission Exhibit Number 856. It shows a bullet that has been fired through a 6.5 mm Mannlicher-Carcano rifle, out of a cartridge similar to that believed to have been used in the John F. Kennedy murder. The bullet was driven through the wrist of a cadaver causing a comminuted fracture of the bones. Note the pronounced deformation of the recovered bullet. This bullet is a typical one recovered from a series of experimental shots. Comparison of this bullet with the mysterious bullet illustrated in Figure 8-1 suggests that the firing tests do not support the official conclusions concerning the role of the mysterious bullet in the assassination event.

second; the skin reduces the velocity of the bullet as it passes through the skin by about 160 feet per second. Thus, the bullet strikes the bone at a velocity of 1000 feet per second minus 160 feet per second, or about 840 feet per second. If the thigh is struck, both skin and muscle mass serve to reduce the velocity before the bullet strikes the femur.

Skin and muscle then inhibit deformation of a bullet that strikes the underlying bone. At velocities over 1000 feet per second, nevertheless, there would be adequate residual velocity left after passage through skin and muscle to insure at least minimally recognizable deformation of a fully metal-jacketed bullet that is not of the armor-piercing variety.

Wilber (1977) has discussed bullet deformation in some detail.

Commission Confusion

On 27 January 1964 an executive (secret) session of the Warren Commission was held. The transcript became available only years after the Report came out; release required the use of the Freedom of Information laws which Congress finally got around to passing.

In a rambling discourse at that session, attorney Rankin admitted that they had a picture of where the bullet entered the back of the late President. The record in the Report and the Hearings shows that the autopsy pathologists were denied by the Committee access to such an important picture.

According to Rankin the bullet entered the President's back below the shoulder blade on the right side and just right of the backbone. This admission in secret session is in accord with the evidence provided by the suit coat and the shirt worn by the President when he was shot. In both garments the entrance holes in the back are 5 or 6 inches below the top of the collar. It is also the position of the entrance hole as marked on the autopsy working sketch by Doctor Boswell. Rankin was perplexed by the location of the entry and admitted that it seemed to be *below* the point of exit if the anterior throat wound were accepted as an exit wound.

A sketch by Wecht (1974) shows the back wound fairly high and to the right of the spinal column (Fig. 8-3). The sketch is presumably based on photographs given him to examine at the National Archives. The sketch seems to be not in accord with the holes in the President's coat and shirt, nor with Rankin's

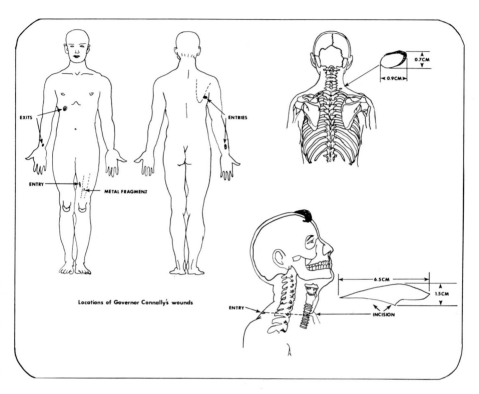

EXITS

ENTRIES

ENTRY

METAL FRAGMENT

0.7CM

0.9CM

Locations of Governor Connally's wounds

6.5CM

1.5CM

ENTRY

INCISION

Figure 8-3. This figure has a pair of diagrams on the left side showing the locations of the nonfatal wounds inflicted on Governor Connally; the diagram on the upper right shows the presumed entrance hole of the nonfatal wound to Kennedy according to the report of Wecht (Wecht and Smith, 1974); and the diagram on the lower right suggests the path for the nonfatal bullet that the Commission claimed went through Kennedy's body. The wounds in the Governor's body line up in such a way as to give a downward angle through him of about 25 degrees. The bullet through Kennedy, at best, is moving nearly horizontal to the ground. The President's death certificate maintained that the nonfatal bullet entered his body in the back at the level of the third thoracic vertebra. The enlarged portion of the upper right figure shows that the bullet hole was oval in outline with a tailing to the right as viewed from behind. This fact indicates that the bullet entered the President's back at an appreciable lateral angle, coming in from the right side as viewed from a position behind the President (Wilber, 1977).

admissions at the executive session of the Commission, nor with the location as given in the death certificate signed by the President's personal physician. The question naturally arises about the technical quality of the photograph that was examined by Wecht. Was adequate information given about viewing distance, orientation of the corpse when the picture was taken, and the position of the photographer when the picture was shot? Were there size references in the picture such as a ruler? What kind of lens was used? What was its focal length? These points all are essential if a useful interpretation of a photograph is to be given.

A much graver question arises. In view of the conflict in the physical evidence that was available, was the photograph examined by Wecht actually authentic? The chain of custody, on the surface at least, appears to have been clouded. Was a foreign photograph substituted for one actually taken at the autopsy but never validated by the pathologists? Serious questions of this sort are inevitably asked in view of the stubborn posture of secrecy that surrounds every scrap of material related to the case. It is obvious that physical evidence would be readily released to scholars if it did support the findings of the Commission as reported. The secrecy, at times verging on the irrational and resulting in depositions by federal officials that are approaching perjury, does, in fact, destroy the basic and crucial conclusions of the Commission.

The Rising Hole

In the attempt to sell the one bullet theory of the nonfatal wounds in the President and Connally, the Commission pushed the posterior thoracic wound higher and higher in order to get it in the neck region and above the hole in the anterior throat region. This so-called neck wound in the Commission's language was referred to by Doctor Humes. "The second wound presumably of entry is that described above in the upper right posterior thorax." For a certified anatomical pathologist the thorax is not the neck. The thorax is anatomically a distinct region of the body below the neck, popularly known as the chest region (*see* Fig. 8-3).

This statement of location of the wound taken in connection with the location of the posterior wound at the level of the third thoracic vertebra as described by the President's personal physician should have been more than adequate to erase forever further reference to a wound in the back of the neck of the President.

The anterior throat wound is still a matter of controversy. Nevertheless, during his testimony before the Commission, Doctor Humes admitted that Doctor Perry of Parkland Hospital told him that the anterior throat wound, before being enlarged for a tracheotomy, was only a few millimeters in diameter. Elsewhere the wound is referred to by Parkland Hospital personnel as "punctate" or round or as an entry wound.

Its interpretation as an exit hole for a bullet going into Kennedy's back at the level of the third thoracic vertebra is untenable. The suggestion that a bone fragment from the base of the President's skull was driven downward and out through the throat area by the force of the head shot is more readily acceptable.

Deformation

One of the questions that arises time and again in discussions of the Kennedy murder is whether the bullet that presumably went through the body of the President, inflicting a nonfatal wound, and then allegedly passed through the chest cavity of Governor Connally, tearing portions of his ribs, smashing through his wrist and lodging in his thigh, could have been the bullet that was later found under mysterious circumstances on a stretcher in Parkland Hospital. Most forensic scientists who have had any experience with gunshot wounds deny that such a bullet, showing absolutely no deformation, could possibly have inflicted the wounds that it was said to have inflicted.

Specter, the lawyer for the Commission asked Colonel Finch, "and could it [the pristine bullet] have been the bullet which inflicted the wound on Governor Connally's right wrist?" Colonel Finck answered without equivocation, "No; for the reason that there are too many fragments described in that wrist."

Later investigators have shown that the fragments of metal in Governor Connally's smashed wrist in no way could be accounted for by the small loss of weight exhibited by the bullet that the Commission claimed wounded him.

Mr. Specter asked Doctor Humes to view the mysterious pristine bullet, which was found on a stretcher left unattended in Parkland Hospital. The question was "could that bullet have gone through or been any part of the fragment passing through President Kennedy's head?" Doctor Humes answered without equivocation, "I do not believe so sir."

Specter pushed the doctor even further and said "and could that missile have made the wound on Governor Connally's right wrist?" Again Doctor Humes said, "I think that that is most unlikely." Doctor Humes then supported his answers by saying that "the x-rays made of the wound in the head of the late President showed fragmentations of a missile. Some fragments we recovered and turned over, as has been previously noted. Also we have x-rays of the fragment of the skull, which was in the region of our opinion exit wound showing metallic fragments." There also was a report from the Parkland Memorial Hospital that referred to the wound in Governor Connally's wrist. It said "small bits of metal were encountered at various levels throughout the wound, and these were, wherever they were identified and could be picked up, and submitted to the Pathology Department for identification and examination."

Doctor Humes then went on to say that "the reason I believe it most unlikely that this missle could have inflicted either of these wounds is that this missile is basically intact; its jacket appears to me to be in the tack [*sic*], and I do not understand how it would possibly have left fragments in either of these locations." This answer seems unequivocal; it was based on logical grounds. It was an answer by the official pathologist for the dead President, an answer that demolished completely any theory that this pristine bullet did, in fact, smash the wrist of Governor Connally. By no stretch of the imagination could the single bullet theory have been accepted in the light of Doctor Humes' clear and unequivocal answer.

In an attempt to salvage what apparently was to be the pristine bullet theory, Specter again asked whether the bullet which went through Kennedy's lower neck or upper chest and then smashed Governor Connally's rib and eventually his wrist and lodged in his thigh could have been the bullet allegedly found on a stretcher in Parkland Hospital. Again Commander Humes said without equivocation, "I think that extremely unlikely." He referred to the entrance wound of the lower midthigh of the Governor and said, "X-rays taken there are described as showing metallic fragments in the bone, which apparently by this report were not removed and are still present in the Governor's thigh. I cannot conceive of where they came from this missile." At that time Representative Ford emphasized, "The missile identified as Exhibit 399." Commander Humes said, "399, sir."

The bullet illustrated in this Commission Exhibit Number 399 could not have caused the wounds in Governor Connally's wrist or the one in his thigh (*see* Fig. 8-1).

With respect to the so-called pristine bullet, which is Commission Exhibit Number 399, Doctor Finck was asked whether he had ever had a chance to examine it. He admitted that just the afternoon of the day during which he was to testify he had had an opportunity to see it. He was then asked by Mr. Specter whether he had any opinion as to whether the bullet could have inflicted the wound in Governor Connally. Doctor Finck said, "This is a bullet showing marks indicating the bullet was fired. The second point is that there was practically no loss of this bullet. It kept its original caliber and dimensions. There was no evidence that any major portion of the jacket was lost, and I consider this as one bullet which possibly could not have gone through the wounds you described." He was then asked by Mr. Specter whether the bullet could possibly have gone through President Kennedy's head and caused the massive head wound. His answer was an unqualified "definitely not." Mr. Specter then said, "And could it have been the bullet which inflicted the wound on Governor Connally's right wrist?" Colonel Finck said, "No; for the reason that there are too many fragments described in that wrist."

In his testimony, Colonel Finck said that he was familiar with the Mannlicher-Carcano 6.5 millimeter rifle and that in his opinion the initial velocity of such a bullet is around 2000 feet per second. Strangely enough he maintained that there would have been little decrease in velocity as a result of a bullet passing through the soft tissues of the President.

The Stretcher Bullet

A rather interesting departure in the Report from the evidence presented by the autopsy team was on page 95 where a discussion of the bullet that presumably wounded Governor Connally took place. An attempt was made to show that the bullet found under mysterious circumstances on a stretcher under the mattress in a corridor in Parkland Hospital was the one that caused the damage. This undamaged bullet presumably left fragments in the Governor's wrist, but was undamaged as far as any external examination is concerned. The statement said, "All these fragments [the fragments found in Governor Connally's wrist wound] were sufficiently small and light so that the nearly whole bullet found on the stretcher could have deposited those pieces of metal as it tumbled through his wrist." How this interesting conclusion could have been drawn from the evidence available is not clear. The conclusion obviously denied the sworn testimony of the autopsy team.

Note the shrewd attempt at beclouding the issue with respect to the single bullet. On page 95 in the Report it was said, "In their testimony, the three doctors who attended Governor Connally at Parkland Hospital expressed independently their opinion that a single bullet had passed through his chest; tumbled through his wrist with very little exit velocity, leaving small metallic fragments from the rear portion of the bullet;

punctured his left thigh after the bullet had lost virtually all its velocity; and had fallen out of the thigh wound." Compare this with the statements made under oath by Doctor Humes and Doctor Finck to the effect that the pristine bullet found in Parkland Memorial Hospital under mysterious circumstances could not have made the wounds in Governor Connally's wrist.

Moreover, the *minimal* velocity for a small projectile to go through human skin, e.g. Connally's thigh skin, is 100 feet per second.

In one part of the Commission Report, it was claimed that the bullet entered Governor Connally's thigh at very low velocity. In fact, in certain parts of the Report and in some commentaries on the Report such as Jim Bishop in his *The Day Kennedy Was Shot,* words are used in such a fashion as to suggest that the bullet merely bored a small hole into the Governor's thigh; consequently, the bullet had very low velocity when it struck. The velocity was said to be so low that after entering the thigh, the bullet fell out backwards and later was found under a mattress on an unattended stretcher found somewhere near an elevator in Parkland Hospital.

On the other hand, that low-velocity bullet caused a wound that was about one centimeter in diameter. A fragment of that bullet was imbedded in the thigh bone. At operation, the fragment was sufficiently imbedded so that the surgeons left it in the bone. It is difficult to reconcile the suggested low velocity of that bullet with the fact that a small fragment ended up imbedded deeply in a hard, long bone.

The location of the wound in the trunk of Governor Connally seemed to change in different portions of the Report. Presumably, this change was necessitated by the requirement that if a single bullet caused the nonfatal wound in President Kennedy and the devastating wounds in Governor Connally, the line of fire somehow had to be straightened out. Be that as it may, according to the surgeon's report, Governor Connally's back wound was just lateral to the right scapula and close to the armpit, or axilla. The bullet then moved around, smashing the rib, and came out below the right nipple. It then smashed his wrist and presumably entered the thigh. The Governor's wounds by themselves line up so that a single bullet clearly caused them. In all probability, the nearly pristine bullet found on a hospital cart had nothing to do with Connally's wounds.

CHAPTER 9

CRITIQUE:
THE HEAD WOUND

THE massive wound to the head of the President was in and of itself sufficient to cause instant death. Biologically the President ceased to exist as an integrated human organism the instant that the bullet destroyed large areas of his brain. Various vegetative functions continued for a period after his death as a human being. It was the monitoring of these residual functions that occupied the doctors at Parkland Memorial Hospital. The details of the head wound, like so much else surrounding this murder, are obscured by secrecy, inadequate records, and obvious tampering (Fig. 9-1).

How many and what kinds of wounds were inflicted on the head of the President?

"The cause of death was due to massive head and brain injury from a gunshot wound of the left temple" (Report, p. 527). So wrote Doctor McClelland in an admission note signed at 4:45 PM 22 November 1963. The autopsy was said to have made no confirmation of this observation by a skilled medical man who was close to the President in the emergency room of Parkland Hospital. In fact, the edited autopsy report was somewhat vague about the left side of the dead President's head. Subsequent secrecy surrounding the autopsy materials suggests that perhaps Doctor McClelland was accurate and that his observation should have been vigorously pursued by investigators of the crime of the century.

What did other doctors on the scene observe? Doctor Carrico described the head wounds as follows. "We opened his shirt and coat and tie and observed a small wound in the anterior lower third of the neck . . . The large skull and scalp wound had been previously observed and was inspected a little more closely. There seemed to be a 4-5 cm. area of avulsion of the scalp and the skull was fragmented and bleeding cerebral and

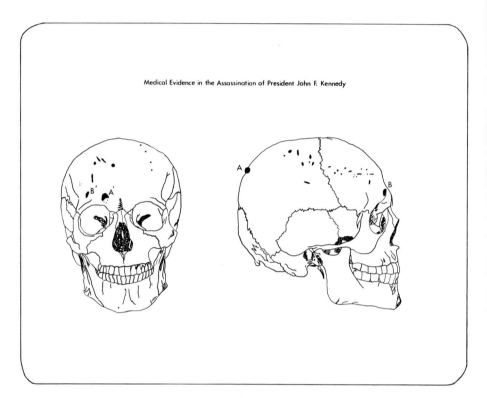

Medical Evidence in the Assassination of President John F. Kennedy

Figure 9-1. This figure shows two diagrams of x-rays of President Kennedy's skull. On the left is a representation of an x-ray taken from the front of the skull. It shows two comparatively large pieces of metal in the head at points A and B. The diagram on the right clarifies the frontal picture; it is taken from the right side of the head. Particle A is shown to be located at the back of the head, probably at the location of the entrance hole. Particle B is shown located over the right eye; as the bullet fragmented that particle moved forward. Others are scattered about the brain substance in a random fashion (Wecht and Smith, 1974; Wilber, 1977).

cerebellar tissue" (Hearings, vol. 6, p. 3).

Doctor Jenkins pointed out that he thought "there was a wound on the left temporal area, right in the hairline and right above the zygomatic process" (Hearings, vol. 6, p. 48).

He was challenged by Specter to the effect that the autopsy report revealed no such wound. Specter could also have admitted that no invasion of the chest cavity was found despite the surgical insertion of chest drainage tubes by skilled surgeons; the autopsy also revealed no brain dissection or bullet track tracing. According to the autopsy report one might conclude that the late President had no endocrine system. Jenkins was not put off by the attempted bullying and Specter went to other matters.

Carrico's further description of the head wound was "the wound that I saw was a large gaping wound, located in the right occipitoparietal area. I would estimate to be about 5 to 7 cm. in size, more or less circular with avulsions of the calvarium and scalp tissue. As I stated before, I believe there was shredded macerated cerebral and cerebellar tissues both in the wounds and on fragments of skull attached to the dura" (Hearings, vol. 6, p. 6).

In the emergency room there was a confirmed observation of a wound to the left side of the head, perhaps a gunshot wound. The autopsy report was claimed by Specter to deny that observation. There were, however, aspects of the autopsy report that indicated some sort of wounding to the left side of the head; strangely, that anatomical area of interest seems not to have been probed with any degree of enthusiasm insofar as the written record reveals.

The FBI report on the autopsy dated 11/26/63 stated that the President's remains were removed from the casket at Bethesda and placed on an autopsy table. The body was wrapped in a sheet; the head had an additional blood saturated sheet wrapped around it. "Following removal of the wrapping, it was ascertained that the President's clothing had been removed and it was also apparent that a tracheotomy had been performed, as well as surgery to the head area, namely, in the top of the skull."*

---

*It has been suggested that ". . . the decision had to be made on the plane to mutilate the President's body at Bethesda Naval Hospital in Washington, D.C. . . ." Allegedly the "surgery" had to be done to deny the observations of the surgeons who treated Kennedy at Parkland Memorial Hospital (Newcomb and Adams, 1974). The process was said to have involved the modification of external wounds and in the removing of bullets and large fragments of bullets from the body. The author has not been able to find persuasive evidence of such modifications from the materials available. The only suggestive evidence in this regard is the report by FBI Special Agents O'Neill and Sibert referring to "surgery to the head."

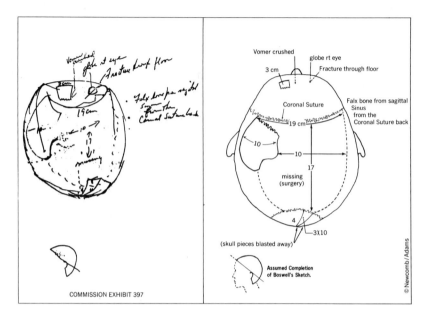

Figure 9-2. The left portion of this figure reproduces Commission Exhibit Number 397, which was drawn by Doctor Boswell, one of the autopsy pathologists, and was printed as part of the Report. The right side of the figure was published by Newcomb and Adams (1975). The poor quality of the original sketch for Commission Exhibit Number 397 is exceeded only by the unacceptable quality of the reproduction of that sketch in the official Report. The left side of this figure shows the level of quality of the drawing which purportedly represents the head wound in one of the most important murder cases of the twentieth century. The right side of this figure is an attempt to clarify the muddled sketch on the left side.

The 3 cm square wound (possibly bone defect) in the area of the left forehead above the eye has never been officially explained. The head wound as described by experienced emergency room surgeons in Dallas seems to be different than the head wounds illustrated in the official autopsy report as published. The question has arisen among competent "noncrankish" forensic scientists, "Did the body arrive in the Naval Hospital for autopsy in essentially the same condition that it left the hands of the emergency room doctors in Dallas?" (From Fred T. Newcomb and P. Adams, Did Someone Alter the Medical Evidence?, *Skeptic, Special Issue No. 9:*27, 1975. Courtesy of publisher.)

No explanation has been made of the "surgery to the head area." Where was it done? When? By whom? Why? The available medical reports from Parkland Memorial Hospital made no mention of surgery on the President other than cutdowns for blood transfusion, a tracheotomy, and the insertion of chest drainage tubes.

The autopsy did not describe any "surgery" to the head.

Either the FBI report in question (file number 89-30 dated 11/26/63 and dictated by Special Agent Francis X. O'Neill, Jr. and Special Agent James W. Sibert on 11/26/630) was false and mistaken or it was true and accurate. If the former, there should have been a clarification of the matter by appropriate consultation among the authors of the report, the pathologists, and the medical personnel from Parkland Memorial Hospital. If the report was accurate, the implications are grave and the report should have been probed exhaustively.

In the absence of a responsible resolution of a serious problem, i.e. surgical modification of the corpse before autopsy, the way was left open to wild speculation about the significance of the FBI contention.*

Facial Injuries

Secret Service Agent Kellerman, who was riding in the front right seat of the presidential limousine when the shooting occurred, swore that the President had no visible injuries to his face when they arrived at Parkland Memorial Hospital (Hearings, vol. 2, p. 82).

At autopsy there was bruising over the right eye. In addition,

---

*According to the FBI report (Commission Document No. 7), near the end of the autopsy a piece of skull 10 by 6.5 cm in size was "brought to Dr. Humes who was instructed that *this had been removed from the President's skull*" (Emphasis added). When, where, by whom, why, and how had this large piece of skull been removed? An x-ray of the piece of bone revealed the presence of metal at one corner. Was this piece the result of the "surgery" that was reported to have been done on the top of the head? Was the FBI report badly worded? If, in fact, it meant what the words seemed to say, who brought in the "removed" piece of skull? From whom did the messenger get the "removed" piece?

the artist's impression of the head wound shows damage in the right occular area. What Kellerman meant when he testified about Kennedy's face, "he was clear," is not apparent. What is apparent is that Kennedy's face was not disfigured upon entry into Parkland Memorial Hospital; it was significantly disfigured at the time of autopsy to an extent that the mortician could not cover over the injury in such a way as to permit an "open coffin."

Evidence from Photography

Olson and Turner (1971), after a careful analysis of photographic evidence in the case of John F. Kennedy's assassination, came to the conclusion that "the exact events of President Kennedy's assassination did not happen as described in the Warren Report." They conceded that, despite a few subsequent disclosures about x-rays of the President's body and notes of executive sessions of the investigating Commission, the only official document available for scholarly study of the assassination was the Report and the volumes of Hearings and Exhibits.

With the passage of time, the value of the suppressed materials decays because of losses, alterations, deliberate destruction, or disappearance of the chain of custody.

More than twenty-five photographers were functioning in Dealey Plaza on the fateful day of 22 November 1963. Nevertheless, interpretation of this well-photographed event has been found inadequate and misleading by an ever increasing number of persons.

The investigating Commission used a color motion picture film by an amateur photographer named Zapruder to sort out the time sequence of the various shots fired at President Kennedy and at Governor Connally. Some film facts may be useful here.

At frame 313 (in the overall sequence of frames in the Zapruder film numbered by the FBI) the head of the President was seen to be wounded. Frames 208 through 224 showed that a highway sign blocked the line of sight from the President to the

Zapruder camera. According to the FBI, frames 166 through 209 showed that the line of sight from the President to the murderer's alleged position in the Texas Book Depository Building was blocked by a live oak tree along the street traveled by the motorcade; for 0.1 second, frame 186, there was a brief gap in the sight barrier created by the tree.

The alleged murder weapon (an Italian, war surplus Mannlicher-Carcano rifle) was demonstrated by the FBI to require no less than 2.3 seconds to fire two successive shots. This time was obtained by test firings at a nonmoving target.

The Zapruder camera was said by FBI reports to have run through the mechanism an average of 18.3 frames per second. Thus it is evident that between two successive shots fired from the claimed assassination rifle, 42 frames of the film passed by the camera lens. As an example, assume the single assassin fired a shot at frame 210; his second shot could not have been fired until frame 252 or subsequent.

Motion picture frame analysis, as well as virtually all competent witnesses, seemed to force the conclusion that the first shot fired struck the President and inflicted a nonfatal wound. The Commission contended that the President did not receive the first shot until frame 210, but he was clearly shot by frame 225 (Report, p. 105).

However, a witness who took six still color pictures of the event (Phil Willis) was seen in the Zapruder film at about frame 183 with his camera raised (Hearings, vol. 7, p. 493). According to Willis, the first shot was fired just before he took the still picture as recorded on motion picture frame 183. According to Willis, ". . . the shot caused me to squeeze the camera shutter, and I got a picture of the President as he was hit with the first shot" (Hearings, vol. 7, p. 493). Careful analysis of the Zapruder film and the Willis slide to confirm the relative positions of Zapruder, Willis, the President, and landmarks revealed that the first shot was fired before frame 202.

Mrs. Kennedy's reaction to the first shot and to her husband's response was described to her and others in the vicinity; her rapid turn toward her injured husband was recorded in

Zapruder frames 195 through 197.

Secret Service Agent Hickey, riding in the automobile behind the President's limousine, was seen to turn rapidly to his right and rise halfway in order to identify the source of the noise; he so testified (Hearings, vol. 18, p. 762). In the Zapruder film at frame 194 he was scanning the crowd to his left; at 195 he began to turn to the right; by frame 207 he was standing halfway and looking hard right.

A still photograph (James Altgens) taken at Zapruder frame 255 (Report, p. 112) revealed Agent Hickey and several other agents looking directly backward toward the Book Depository.

The President himself, by frames 225 through 230 (as he moved from behind the sight-blocking road sign), reacted strongly to a wound, leaning forward, hands clutching at the area of his neck and chin, elbows elevated to chin level. Early frames, 194 through 206, showed movements by the President forward and leftward by about 6 inches. These movements occurred before the Zapruder filming was blocked by the highway sign. At frame 204 the President was turned virtually straight forward. His right arm was pulled inside the car and bent up to his neck. Witnesses described these movements that were seen in frames 194 through 206 (Hearings, vol. 7, p. 473; vol. 6, p. 273).

Governor Connally and his wife were forceful and unequivocal about holding that the first shot hit Kennedy, the second, Connally. The Governor studied exhaustively enlargements of the Zapruder frames made by *Life* magazine; he picked frame 234 as the frame in which he was shot.

A minute in the administrative file of the Warren Commission, apparently 21 April 1964, recorded Connally's contention. "He (Connally) felt the President might have been hit by frame 190. He heard only two shots and felt sure that the shots he heard were the first and third shots. He is positive that he was hit after he heard the first shot: i.e. by the second shot, and by that shot only."

An unpublished Warren Commission FBI report indicated that Secret Service Agent Howlett, after a study in depth of the 8 mm movie film of the assassination "advised that it had been ascertained from the movies that President Kennedy was struck with the first and third shots fired by the assassin, while Governor Connally was struck with the second shot" (National Archives, Warren Commission File No. 5, 117).

From photographic time analysis alone, one is compelled to deny the Warren Commission single bullet theory. This denial is supported by competent witnesses as indicated.

Wound ballistic evidence developed elsewhere in this book further demonstrates the unacceptability of the single bullet theory.

Location of the Late President's Head Wound

A critique of the information given about the head wound that killed President Kennedy was influenced by reports from the secret panel of pathologists and others called together in February 1968 by then Attorney General Ramsey Clark.*

Allegedly the panel examined the photographs and x-rays taken at the time of autopsy; there was no indication that photomicrographs of the wounds were studied; the brain itself was kept hidden from the panel.

The panel reported that an entry hole existed in the back of the President's skull 10 cm above the external occipital protuberance; that is a distance of almost 4 inches. The autopsy pathologists officially reported the hole to be a little above and about 1 inch to the right of the external occipital protuberance (Nichols, 1973).

If the secret panel's observation was correct, then the entrance hole in the President's skull was almost on the top of his head, if they measured the distance along the curve of the skull. If the measurement was a straight vertical distance above the protuberance, the entrance hole was almost a glancing one.

Could there have been two holes of entrance in the skull? Could there have been one hole seen and located at autopsy by the doctors who never saw the pictures and another seen in the

---

*It is interesting to note that one of the pathologists involved in the panel later testified that an exhumation and autopsy of Mary Jo Kopechne would be of no value in revealing information that might have been missed.

pictures by a panel who never saw the body?

Discrepancies of such magnitude between an "official" autopsy report and the photographs of the material being described by pathologists in the autopsy report raise grave and valid questions. Was the head described in the autopsy report the same one that was illustrated in a batch of unverified pictures? On a flat photograph, how did the panel measure curved distances? Were there size reference marks or calibration scales in the photographs? What was the position of the body or the body part when it was photographed? What exposure data and developing data were recorded for each picture? What was the proper viewing distance for each photograph?

Did the Warren Commission refuse, in a most inexplicable way, to review the photographs and x-rays made at the autopsy because they had suspicions of their authenticity but were loath to follow up on the matter?

In a photograph presumably of the President's brain, the secret panel saw a rectangular object (really a body giving a four-sided parallelogram outline as viewed from the photograph) which had a gray brown cast to it. Its size was 0.14 by 0.20 centimeter. In no part of the autopsy report or the supplement to it did the pathologists mention this object. If they examined the brain and photographed it, how could they have missed the odd body in the brain? Why was it not discussed in the protocol?

In addition, a mistlike path of metal particles was seen in the soft tissues of the President's neck in an x-ray examined by the panel. No such trail of metal was reported by the doctor, a radiologist who read the x-ray films during the autopsy.

A copper-clad bullet passing between muscle masses and avoiding all bone en route virtually never leaves a streak of metal particles behind. Very soft lead unjacketed bullets may do so, but it is unusual under the circumstances described for the nonfatal wound track in the President.

These discrepancies call into question the competence of the published draft of the autopsy report. In the face of admitted destruction by fire of notes made at the autopsy and of other related papers, this strange oversight can readily be given an unfavorable interpretation.

There is clear and persistent evidence that the autopsy itself was "managed"; the report of the autopsy was edited, modified, and otherwise adjusted so that its scientific value is difficult to judge. Fundamental materials directly related to the competence of the autopsy report (specimens, photographs, x-rays) were compromised and contaminated by official misbehavior (lying as to status, hiding, losing, denying existence) to such a degree as to support an investigation of felonious action. Of greater concern is the high probability that these materials no longer have probative or historical value as a result of the actions of numerous federal officials.

Experimental Head Shots

Experimental studies of head injuries caused by bullets indicate that for a given caliber of bullet, the damage is related directly to the velocity of the bullet that strikes the head (Clemedson et al., 1973). As a general rule, low-velocity bullets produce a more or less tubular wound passage having a diameter close to that of the bullet. High-velocity bullets, on the other hand, tend to produce a wound passage that rapidly increases in diameter as the bullet moves through the head. High-velocity ammunition also produces shock waves and "a particularly powerful pressure wave effect" (Clemedson et al., 1973). High-velocity bullets also tend to fragment. The entrance wound caused by high-velocity ammunition in the head is usually close to the diameter of the bullet.

With high-velocity bullets, bone fragments act as secondary missiles and contribute to the damage; projectile fragments are common with high-velocity bullets and cause additional damage.

The size of exit wounds of high-velocity bullets varies directly with the impact velocity of the bullet. Pressures produced in brain tissue by the shock wave created by high-velocity bullets vary approximately with the square of the velocity of the bullet. Bullet mass has little significance.

If this sort of information is used to evaluate the head wound of the President, it seems probable that the damage was caused by a bullet having a velocity significantly higher than is found in the usual commercial cartridge available as war surplus items for the 6.5 mm Mannlicher-Carcano rifle. Either a special hand-loaded cartridge was used or the head wound was caused by another rifle. Reloaded 6.5 mm Mannlicher-Carcano rifle cartridges have been available in which the military-style fully jacketed bullet was pulled out and replaced by a hunting-style bullet with an exposed lead nose.

Experimental studies have indicated that when a bullet enters the skull at right angles to the surface, the diameter of the entrance hole produced is smaller than the caliber of the bullet (Tamaska, 1964). The difference is usually several tenths of a millimeter; but it has been observed to be as much as a millimeter. The explanation seems to be that live bone is extremely elastic; it opens up to permit the bullet to pass through and form an entrance hole; it springs back to a smaller diameter hole once the bullet has passed through. The difference in diameter is said to be a regularly occurring event (Tamaska, 1964). It is therefore probable that a hole of entrance measured in live skull has been made by a bullet with a diameter of 0.1 to 1.0 millimeter larger than the hole.

The entrance hole in the back of Kennedy's skull was said to have been compatible with having been made by a 6.5 mm bullet; it was also compatible, perhaps even more probable, with having been made by a 7 mm bullet.

Entrance holes in skin caused by distant shots also tend to be smaller in diameter than the bullet causing them. The skin is elastic and pulls together as the bullet passes through it.

The Brain

An essential aspect of the examination of the fatal wound to President Kennedy's head would have been an examination of the brain itself, which was preserved in formaldehyde. Indeed, the official Armed Forces Institute of Pathology *Autopsy Manual* specifies that such examination will be done and describes in detail how it is to be carried out. When they go through brain tissue, bullets leave a track. Generally the brain is hardened in formaldehyde after it is taken out of the head. After the brain tissue hardens satisfactorily, one or two weeks in formaldehyde, it is then carefully dissected in order to follow the path that the bullet or bullet fragments may have taken.

According to records in the National Archives, the brain of the President was in existence a year and one-half after President Kennedy was murdered. At that time, Admiral Burkley indicated in a memorandum the transfer of various materials to the National Archives; various autopsy materials including the brain and a set of microscopic slides made after the autopsy were included in this document transferring materials to the National Archives. Admiral Burkley was Kennedy's personal physician.

Strangely enough, since that time the brain and the slides are said to have disappeared. Officials at the National Archives claim no knowledge of the whereabouts of these vital bits of evidence. Where are they? No one in authority admits to any knowledge concerning the whereabouts of the brain and the microscope slides. No one in authority has permitted competent, serious, biomedical scholars to examine autopsy materials in the way they deserve to be examined scientifically.

Despite the fact that the slides and the preserved brain have disappeared, there were some large photographs allegedly made of the late President's brain. In the front part of the right cerebral hemisphere of the brain in one of the photographs available, there was (as indicated previously) a dark brownish black object that had a white glistening effect. This object measured about 13 by 20 millimeters, about 3/4 by 1 1/2 inches. The object could have been larger than what was shown in the photograph because the brain material around it seemed to hide the borders of this unidentified object. Despite the fact that some thirty-five pieces of metal were accounted for in the President's head (many of these no bigger than a grain of sand, but they were accounted for), this large and obvious object was ignored at the original autopsy and in the superficial description of the formalin-fixed brain of the President. This latter description was part of the supplement to the basic autopsy report filed by the military pathologists.

What was this strange object? Was it the remains of a hemorrhage caused by the gunshot wounds? Was it a piece of metal or a respectable chunk of a bullet fragment? Was it a brain tumor or some kind of malformation in the blood vessels in that part of the brain? It seems proper to exclude a hemorrhage caused by a gunshot wound. If such a hemorrhage did exist, it is inconceiveable that the pathologists who performed the autopsy would not have recorded that fact. Because of the size of this object shown in the photograph, it is difficult to accept the view that the three doctors who performed the autopsy failed to observe it.

There is one conclusion that can be made concerning this particular object, whatever it might have been: Reference to this object was purposely and willfully omitted from the report. The reason for this omission cannot be stated on the basis of the evidence available.

If this mysterious object in the brain of the President was a bullet or a fragment of a bullet, where then did the bullet come from or where did the fragment come from? Did this particular object indicate that there was another gunman and that President Kennedy received two shots to the head instead of one?

The Left Rear Head Wound

There was another odd aspect to President Kennedy's autopsy report. This peculiarity was exposed as a result of an examination of the autopsy photographs by several groups. These photographs, said by the National Archives to have been made at the autopsy of President Kennedy, showed a loose flap of skin on the left side of the back part of the late President's head. Careful examination of the entire twenty-six volumes of the Warren Commission publication failed to reveal anywhere that this wound was mentioned. It was not mentioned in the autopsy report.

The loose flap of skin could have been the exit wound of a bullet or fragment. The condition of the underlying bone was not revealed by the photograph. If indeed this skin flap represented an exit wound, one is then faced with the possibility of a shot coming from in front of the President and exiting rearward.

An entrance shot in the left temple, as Doctor McClelland testified, could also have caused such an exit wound in the back of the head.

Momentum

Much is currently being made of a so-called snapping backward of the head of the late President as allegedly revealed by a careful analysis of the Zapruder film. Commentators on the Warren Commission Report and defenders of the Report are involved in evaluating the head snap. It is claimed that the momentum of a bullet coming from in front of the President pushed his head back at a high velocity. Defenders of the Report talk about "jet effects" that could explain the observation. Even if the observation had some validity, it tells nothing about the origin of the head shot or its energy; in fact, assuming the observation is true, it is irrelevant to the whole matter.

It is the basic premise in physics that the momentum of a system consisting of a moving object impacting a stationary object is the same before and after the impact. The system composed of the 6.5 mm Mannlicher-Carcano bullet impacting the head of the late President Kennedy had the following physical relationships. The presumed weight of the bullet was 160 grains. The estimated impact velocity of the bullet at 60 yards was 1900 feet per second. Thus, 160 grains times 1900 feet per second equals 304,000 foot grains per second. Divide that by 7000 grains (number of grains in a pound) and the result is 43 foot pounds per second, the momentum of the bullet in impact.

The momentum of the Kennedy-bullet system would also have been 43 foot pounds per second (conservation of momentum). Assume a 170 pound body weight with all the momentum transferred to the whole body. Then 43 divided by

170 equals 0.25 foot per second of velocity imparted to the body, an amount less than 10 percent of the speed of a walking man and no more than 1 percent of the speed of a running man.

One may argue that only the head was involved in the momentum system considered in the Zapruder film. Assume that the head makes up about 20 percent of the total body weight; then 170 divided by 5 equals 34. Further, 43 divided by 34 equals 1.1 feet per second, or no more that 50 percent of the velocity of a walking man or 5 percent of the speed of a running man.

It is obvious that the so-called "push" (as a result of examination by critics of the Zapruder home-style movie) that the bullet is said to have given to the President's head is a nonexistent physical phenomenon. Irregular feeding of the film through the camera, motion of the limousine, or some other unidentified factor may explain what was thought to have been seen in the film. It is clear, however, that there was no "knockdown" or other kind of "pushing" of the President by a bullet. Basic energy relations permit no such explanation and give absolutely no support to the idea of a shot into the head from the front.

Whether a shot from in front of the President did go into his head may be uncertain. It is certain that the answer of head snapping as a result of bullet impact cannot be used to support a conclusion about where any bullet came from.

Alvarez, a Nobel prize winning physicist, has reported the results of an examination of the Zapruder film (1976). He tested experimentally the backward "snap" of the President's head and body immediately after the shot to the head. His experiments and theoretical considerations of momentum supports the conclusion that the President was shot in the head from behind. Alvarez stated, "I believe that our experimental demonstration of retrograde recoil in head-like objects will convince most people that the laws of physics do not require a second assassin to have been firing at the President from the 'grassy knoll' ahead of the car." A footnote to the report by Alvarez (1976, note 13) indicates that the suggestions of a hunting-style bullet having been used for the head shot is not frivolous.

The head-snapping controversy does illustrate the mischief caused by the "managed" medicolegal investigation of President Kennedy's murder. Had a competent autopsy been done and the results published openly, completely, and without mutilation, much of the unfortunate response to the Warren Commission investigation might have been avoided. Deceit at every level of government spawns more damage than the matter the deceit was supposed to cover up.

Angle of the Head Shot

Lieutenant Colonel Pierre Finck was called to testify on the head wound. Colonel Finck had been head of the Wound Ballistics Branch at the Armed Forces Institute of Pathology and had reviewed hundreds of cases of gunshot wounds from all agencies of the Department of Defense. He was asked whether the President received the head wound from behind or from what direction. He testified that the small hole in the President's skull was an entry hole and consequently the President had been shot from behind. He was then asked by Mr. Specter at what angle from behind was he shot? Colonel Finck answered honestly, "In my opinion, the angle can be determined only approximately due to the fact that wound of entrance is fairly small and could give enough precision in the determination of the path, but the dimension of the wound of exit . . . is so large that we can only give an approximate angle. In my opinion, the angle was within 45° on a horizontal plane" (Hearings, vol. 2, p. 380). In other words, the angle could not have been more than 45 degrees above the horizontal but it could have been virtually any other angle down to almost horizontal, according to Colonel Finck.

This answer was understandable and honest, because if one were to have projected through the entrance hole into the exit wound and then moved the projected line through the possible revolutions delimited by the size of the exit wound, one then had the option of selecting an angle anywhere from almost horizontal to 45 degrees above horizontal. This fact was dramatically illustrated when it was learned from Colonel Finck that the greatest dimension of the exit wound was 13 cm (about 5 inches).

In discussing the pristine bullet, Colonel Finck gave answers that were confusing. Specter asked that, since the weapon being dealt with had a muzzle velocity in excess of 2000 feet per second and since the automobile carrying the President was 50 yards away from the muzzle of the gun, would there have been any significant loss of velocity over the 50 yard range? Colonel Finck said, "At this range, a bullet at this velocity loses very little velocity, and keeps upon impact a large amount of kinetic energy."

According to the ballistics tables published in the 1975 edition of *Gun Digest,* the 6.5 millimeter Carcano cartridge has a bullet weighing 156 grains. The muzzle velocity in feet per second is 2000; at 100 yards, the muzzle velocity is 1810 feet per second. The muzzle energy is 1386 foot pounds; at 100 yards, the muzzle energy is 1135 foot pounds. One can interpolate to the 50-yard point and the following results are obtained. The velocity at 50 yards then would be about 1900 feet per second; this velocity would result in a calculated loss of 5 percent of the muzzle velocity. The muzzle energy compared with the energy at 100 yards gives the following interpolation. The energy at 50 yards would be 1285 foot pounds, or a reduction from the muzzle energy at 50 yards of about 7 percent.

Further questioning about the pristine bullet found on a stretcher at Parkland Memorial Hospital elicited the admission from Doctor Finck that he could not conclude that the mysterious bullet in question could have caused the nonfatal wounds to Kennedy and to Connally. The lack of deformation and the minuscule loss of weight, in his estimation, precluded that bullet as the causative agent for the nonfatal wounds.

A Final Word

The available evidence leaves one in a quandry with respect to the head wounds. An entrance wound seems to have been made somewhere in the rear of the President's skull; the bullet causing that hole came from behind. The precise direction is unknown; possible lateral and horizontal angles are too great to be helpful.

This entry hole was never located reliably. According to testimony, the hole was said to vary from one place to another in the back of the skull by a difference of 4 inches.

A bullet hole to the left temple was seen by competent surgeons upon close examination of the moribund President's head. Nothing more is known of that wound. An exitlike flap was seen in pictures of the head in the occipital area; nothing more is known of that hole.

Alleged "surgery" done to the top of the President's head has never been explained. The FBI report of this surgery did suggest strongly that some sort of modification was made to the President's remains before the pathologists began their work. Who? Why? Where? How? There are no answers.

The mysterious body seen imbedded in the President's brain, as revealed in photographs examined by a secret panel of experts convened by former Attorney General Ramsey Clark, is unexplained. The discovery of this body reflects adversely on the quality of the original autopsy examination.

In sum, there is evidence of a shot to the head from somewhere behind the President. There is also evidence of a shot from at least one other direction into the head. The end result seems inevitable: More than one person fired at and hit the late President Kennedy in the head. If the available evidence can be believed, the Mannlicher-Carcano rifle found after the shooting was used in the crime but it was not the only gun involved. Whether Oswald fired the rifle cannot be decided on the basis of the head wound.

CHAPTER 10

CONCLUSIONS OF A
FORENSIC SCIENTIST

The Commission Format

$\mathbf{A}$ BASIC flaw in the overall operation of the President's Commission on the Assassination of President Kennedy was its total commitment to the adversary system format. The "hearings" were carried out seemingly in the only way that lawyers understand.

Unfortunately the format used resulted in a one-legged monster, out of balance and disoriented. The air of the Hearings and of the deposition sessions was clearly prosecutorial. There were the good guys and the bad guys in the cast of characters. The former were those who testified in favor of the prosecution; the latter, those who presented testimony against the Commission's predetermined conclusions.

The absolute elimination of any semblance of cross-examination during the Hearings virtually insured that a distorted, confused, disjointed, and slanted version of the facts would emerge. The adversary system in the courts, despite pious disclaimers, is not designed to reveal the truth; it is designed for the purpose of winning cases in court. Lawyers use the system, as their law professors train them, to win convictions or acquittals as the case may be. The whole truth is kept out of the record, if need be, in order to make one's own case stronger. The cross-examination procedure in part brings about a balance and helps to modulate the nefarious results of an unrestrained adversary system in operation.

In the Commission Hearings, one witnessed all the evils of the adversary system without the modulating effects of cross-examination. The result was, of course, a disastrous final Report in which one reads of witnesses being harrassed and bullied, data suppressed, the Commission's own experts impeached or ignored, and a ridiculous conclusion generated, later to be supported in challenge by a consistent plan of villifying independent scholars who presumed to question any segment of the Report.

The suppression of Documents and Exhibits, the editing and censoring of fundamental data, e.g. the autopsy report, and the twisting of evidence to fit a preconceived conclusion illustrates how the "hearing" format is conducive to hiding the truth.

When the Commission maneuverings are recognized as having been carried out by lawyers with no technical competence in subjects critical to the investigation (ballistics, biology, forensic medicine, firearms, forensic science generally), it is understandable that an inadequate report was the result.

What is not understandable or forgivable is the failure of the Commission itself, also composed of persons who were technically incompetent for the job they undertook, to engage the services of forensic science experts of international stature to advise and consult with them. The bulk of such experts was then and is now in the United States. All would have made themselves available to search for the truth of the tragic murder of John F. Kennedy. All were ignored by the Commission and its staff.

The Hypothetical Question

In courts of law, a hypothetical question is often proposed to an expert witness so that he can use the statements made and render an opinion based on the assumption that the statements are true and factual. At best a hypothetical question is a weak device in a court trial because the entire question is so artificial. It just does not picture the whole factual truth. Lawyers present biased narratives and, of course, neglect to include in the question facts which are inconvenient for their side. A skillful lawyer can readily draw out from an honest, conscientious expert an answer that misleads (Moenssens, Moses, and Inbau, 1973).

The use of the hypothetical question in an adversary encounter in court is bad enough unless rigorously controlled by the court. In a hearing that is presumed to be undertaken for the sole purpose of revealing the truth, the use of the hypothetical question is deceitful and despicable. It is misleading and can be thought of as nothing more than a cheap trick that has no place in a commission probing for the truth under any circumstances.

The lawyers on the staff of the Warren Commission used the hypothetical question as a device to twist the direct testimony of key witnesses such as the doctors from Parkland Hospital who treated the President *in extremis* and the pathologists who performed the autopsy. There was no excuse then and no excuse can be dredged up now for the shabby trick of using the hypothetical question to obfuscate and contort the results of the Warren Commission's endeavor.

The Commission itself included enough lawyers so that one cannot excuse that body on the basis of ignorance. There is clear and unequivocal evidence from the Commission Hearings themselves that factual evidence presented by such experts as Doctor Perry of Parkland Hospital was turned around using the hypothetical question as the instrument.

Strangely enough, Doctor McClelland, who stated in his report of the President's final minutes that the "cause of death was due to massive head and brain injury from a gunshot wound of the left temple," was not badgered into retracting that written report and actually reaffirmed it during the course of his testimony before the Commission lawyers. In the final Report of the Commission his testimony was completely ignored, as if it simply did not exist.

The hypothetical question ploy as it was used by the Warren Commission lawyers raises a grave question of the competence and appropriateness of having lawyers in charge of a search for the truth. American lawyers are by and large so hammered into the adversary system frame of thought that serious scholars may well question their ability or desire to reach objective truth.

Perhaps investigating commissions should use the symposium format with question periods after each presentation to break the strangle hold that lawyers seem to have on the mechanisms for uncovering the truth in "official hearings."

The Death Certificate

A death certificate of sorts was filed for the President's body. Its legality and propriety are open to serious question. It was signed by Rear Admiral George Gregory Burkley, physician to the President, and was dated 23 November 1963. Aside from the peculiarity of the death certificate signed by a doctor who was neither the autopsy pathologist nor the one who treated the deceased in his last illness, there was information on it about the wounds that is pertinent.

The certificate stated that the President was "struck in the head by an assassin's bullet and a second wound occurred in the posterior back at about the level of the third thoracic vertebra." The third thoracic vertebra is in the upper chest region; it is not in the neck.

The head wound was described. "The wound was shattering in type causing a fragmentation of the skull and avulsion of three particles of the skull at the time of the impact, with the resulting maceration of the right hemisphere of the brain."

Fragmentation of the skull and maceration of the brain are compatible with a hunting-type bullet wound of the head, not with a wound produced at 60 yards from a medium-velocity rifle with a metal-jacketed bullet.

No mention was made in the death certificate of the anterior throat wound. Was this an oversight? Burkley seemed to have been in careful control of matters throughout the assassination episode. It is reasonable to conclude that his failure to mention the anterior throat wound in the death certificate was calculated.

No Pictures

A significant amount of confusion and misunderstanding connected to the final Report of the Commission was created by the persistent, wrongheaded, and irrational refusal of the Commission to view the illustrations made at the autopsy and indeed to permit the very doctors who generated the illustrations to have access to them. This posture of the Commission cannot be excused or justified in any way. Individually and as a group, the Commission advertised its incompetence and suggested its own lack of integrity (individually and collectively) by the suppression of the basic data collected at the autopsy. Armed Forces directives ordered that x-rays and photographs be attached to autopsy reports as essential parts of those documents.

A cogent comment was made by Doctor Humes on page 8 of his handwritten draft of the autopsy (Commission Exhibit No. 397). In referring to the massive head wound he stated, "The complexity of these fractures and the fragments thus produced tax satisfactory verbal description and are better appreciated in photographs and [deleted] roentgenograms which are prepared." Apparently the Commission had no interest in fully appreciating the head wounds or any other wounds for that matter. In addition they seemed doggedly determined that no competent scientists would be given a clear appreciation of the wounds.

During Doctor Humes' testimony before the Commission, the lawyer Specter attempted to suggest that photographs and x-rays were unusual procedures in autopsies. Humes made it quite clear that the contrary was true. It had no effect on the Commission and they continued to discuss complicated matters of wounding on the basis of silly artist's cartoons drawn by a hapless Navy enlisted man who had never seen the wounded body nor any of the photographs of that body.

In passing, it is appropriate to mention that some of the world's outstanding medical artists practice in the United States. In Baltimore, just thirty miles from Washington, D.C., there are two outstanding training centers for medical artists. If the delicate stomachs of the Commission might have been upset by the actual photographs, there was no reason that they did not engage the services of competent medical artists who could have produced from the original photographs and x-rays anatomically precise color illustrations devoid of gruesomeness.

(How an x-ray can be gruesome is obscure, but lawyers and politicians do have obscure ways of thought at times.) The fact that they failed to do so calls to mind *res ipsa loquitur*. The thing speaks for itself and shouts dereliction.

Silencing

According to the *New York Times* of 6 December 1963 the military medical officers who carried out the autopsy procedures maintained that they had been ordered not to talk about the case. Personal acquaintances of these officers confirm the fact that some sort of potent "silencing" maneuver was used against these men, for whatever the reason. Even after the final volumes of the Report were distributed to the public, the military pathologists refused to discuss with scientific colleagues the technical aspects of their work.

In part this silencing may explain why some of the technical aspects of the postmortem examination were so inadequate.

In sworn testimony in criminal court (State of Louisiana v. Clay Shaw, 1969) Doctor Finck explained why the pathologists at J.F. Kennedy's autopsy did not dissect out and visualize the bullet track of the back-throat wound over which there has been so much controversy. In answer to direct examination, Colonel Finck admitted that an Army general, whose name he could not remember, stated that he was "in charge" at the autopsy scene. He also admitted that the general was not a pathologist. He further revealed that "at the end of the autopsy we were specifically told — as I recall it, it was by Admiral Kenney, the Surgeon General of the Navy — this is subject to verifications — we were specifically told not to discuss the case." As the questioning under oath progressed, Doctor Finck asserted, "I did not dissect the track in the neck . . . We didn't remove the organs of the neck." With these admissions made, the attorney questioning Doctor Finck finally had to appeal to the judge to get an answer *why* the wound track was not dissected. The answer from Colonel Finck was "as I recall I was told not to, but I don't remember by whom." He further admitted that they were "told" to examine the head and chest cavity and apparently not much else. Later Finck spelled out the name of the admiral who had ordered the pathologists not to discuss the autopsy; it was K-i-n-n-e-y.

It is obvious that administrative interference with the full development of the case began certainly as early as the actual autopsy dissections and perhaps even earlier. The scene was set for such interference by the fact that the pathologists were military men in uniform. Had the autopsy pathologists been civilians of stature, no such unethical and abominable interference would have been tolerated. Was that why no civilian experts were called in as observers of the autopsy?

More importantly, however, the orders not to do certain procedures were contrary to published directives of the Armed Forces Institute of Pathology as expressed in the official *Autopsy Manual*. The situation, then, was not carelessness or panic; it was the issuance of unlawful orders by senior officers of the military services in matters of grave national concern. Such behavior merits a general court martial.

The Chain of Custody

The chain of custody of the critical x-rays and photographs that were part of the autopsy protocol was not complete. The pathologists did not see the photographs and hence could not verify their authenticity. The custodians of the evidence who could be identified had no technical or medical competence to associate the photographs with any given subject. Thus, from the point of view of authenticity, the photographs said to have been made at the autopsy of President Kennedy (now on file in the National Archives) are in limbo.

After a vague period when the exact location of the photographs was as obscure as how they got there, the x-rays and photographs appeared in the records of the Archivist of the United States in April 1965. A strange and (to scholars and scientists at least) outrageous provison was attached to their use. Only such scholars as might be approved by the Kennedy family lawyers could have access to the x-rays and photographs. Until that time it was unthinkable that the family of a murder victim had any control directly or indirectly over items of evidence in the case.

Consultation with several outstanding attorneys and one judge indicates that neither the photographs nor the x-rays could have been entered into evidence in any court in the land. Had Oswald not been murdered and had he been brought to trial, the x-rays and the photographs were so badly contaminated as evidence that they could not have become part of the case.

There is also serious doubt that the autopsy protocol would have been admitted in evidence in any trial. It had been censored; it was incomplete; new evidence and internal peculiarities threw its accuracy into question; it was the result of inadequate procedures that violated basic principles clearly outlined in the official military *Autopsy Manual*; significant technical data were made unavailable to the pathologist who presumably wrote the published version; and the critical data were known to have been in existence at the time they were kept from the pathologists.

The mysterious pristine bullet said to have caused the nonfatal wounds in Kennedy and Connally was found under circumstances that would deny its admission as evidence in any court. Its later history was vague enough to deny it as acceptable evidence.

At this late date, the contaminated evidence cannot be purged and rendered acceptable in court. It, therefore, is apparent that a new look at the J.F. Kennedy murder and the Commission Report on it can do little to bring to justice still-living persons who may have been involved in the murder and its cover-up. The obfuscation endeavors have been effective in that regard.

Nevertheless, a complete reexamination of the incident is warranted to set straight the *historical record* so that the tragedy may teach us how to obviate future dilemmas of this sort.

Lost, Strayed, or Stolen?

During the time Ramsey Clark was Attorney General of the

United States, Doctor Cyril Wecht, Coroner of Allegheny County in Pennsylvania and a distinguished forensic scientist, was able to look at some previously secret medical data connected with the murder of John F. Kennedy. Doctor Wecht found that important microscope slides of tissues taken at the autopsy were not among the case materials in the National Archives. Moreover, the preserved brain of the murdered President had disappeared from the Archives although it appeared to have been "logged in" at a previous date.

These losses were serious, especially since the brain had never been dissected.

Later, authorities at the Archives claimed to have "found" a metal container marked "gross material." There is no public record available of any competent, independent scientist having seen the "gross material." Why? Is there something in the container that important government officials fear to have exposed to the light of day? Is there perhaps a bullet buried in the formalin-hardened brain?

The secret panel of scientific examiners brought together by Ramsey Clark to look at some of the autopsy photographs reported an unidentified object in the brain substance, rectangular in outline, as revealed in one of the photographs. The panel never saw the brain itself. The original autopsy pathologists apparently never saw the object, or at least they never made any notation of record about it. Was their observation of it, if made, edited out of the published report by the pathologists' superiors?

If there is nothing of substance hidden away among the remaining autopsy materials associated with the John F. Kennedy murder, is not the compulsive secrecy about the materials somewhat irrational?

After over a decade of peculiar behavior and responses by central government officials when asked that adequate scientific study be made of whatever autopsy materials are still in existence, it now seems clear that these materials contain information that could answer some or all of the following questions.

• Were there additional bullets or bullet fragments in tissues or organs not previously reported?

- Do photographs and actual specimens demonstrate that the conclusions of the Warren Commission, insofar as they involve autopsy material, are unwarranted?
- Were the autopsy pathologists ordered to do only a superficial examination of the body and did they supress, under orders, matters of crucial importance to the diagnosis? Did higher officials delete important information from the autopsy report?
- Have materials that were part of the complete autopsy record been "lost" or destroyed? If so, when? Under whose custody were they at the time of disappearance? What were the attending circumstances?
- Was there something of a grave nature having widespread implications that is being suppressed? Were the actions and behavior of one or more federal officials of national stature of such a nature as to impel other officials over the years to conceal these activities by elaborate devices?
- Are the photographs and x-rays of the autopsy, reportedly held by the National Archives, the original ones? Have there been substitutions, mutilations, retouchings, or destructions?

If these questions have a clear negative answer, the justification of the secrecy is not apparent. If any of these questions has a positive answer, the invoked secrecy is then part of a larger criminal act.

Custody of the Remains

Newcomb and Adams (1975) pose some thoughtful questions about the medicolegal aspects of the Kennedy murder. They point out that the main evidence in the case was never directly examined by the Commission. As any forensic scientist knows, the body itself speaks and reveals a wealth of information concerning a violent death, if the right questions are asked and the resulting answers recorded faithfully. That action was never taken by the Commission.

The serious problem is the custody of the body of the late President from the time it left the emergency room, spirited away illegally by federal officials, and the time that the autopsy pathologists first had an opportunity to view it. Was the body in the same condition when first seen by the pathologists who performed the autopsy in Maryland as it was when it was last seen by the doctors who attempted to save the President's life in Dallas? The chain of custody is obscure.

The trip from Andrews Air Force Base to the Naval Hospital at Bethesda took about forty-five minutes. What happened during that time? Who was in immediate charge of the body? Where was the receipt system for the body showing all the changes of custody and accounting for all the time between Dallas and Bethesda? The Commission seemed not interested, which is a rather strange posture for lawyers who know the details that a court would demand in order to establish the fact of a crime.

The clothing of the President was presumably removed in Dallas. By whom? What happened to it? The available record indicates that the pathologists did not have the items of clothing available for reference during the actual anatomical examination. Indeed, the pathologists saw the clothing (according to the Record) only a few minutes before they were asked to testify before the Commission months after the event. Such a situation is contrary to military directives and routinely accepted forensic pathology standards of acceptable performance.

What happened to the body brace and Ace bandage that the President wore?

These questions are of importance if for no other reason than to clarify the supplemental autopsy report, which includes a sketchy description of the microscopic examination of some of the tissues taken from the body. The presence of even a beginning of tissue or cellular decomposition or autolysis was denied for every tissue section that was reported. It is unusual to find all cells and tissues "essentially normal" in samples taken from a body that has been dead a number of hours and has not been specially cooled or otherwise treated to inhibit decomposition.

The anterior throat wound was such a confusing factor that it needs a thorough reexamination. The Commission seemed to reflect the view in the Report that the anterior wound was cut out or excised in the process of inserting an air tube into the moribund President's windpipe, just below the voice box. Doctor Perry, who performed the operation, and the surgeons who observed the manipulation reported that Doctor Perry had "extended" the existing hole by cutting across the lower part of it. When that wound was described by the pathologists in the autopsy report, the impression given was of a rather long slash with gaping edges that were irregular in appearance. How did the wound change in appearance from Dallas to Bethesda? Perhaps the explanation is straightforward; but the Commission seemed not interested. Why were the edges of the wound in the anterior throat as seen by the pathologists not approximated in an attempt to reconstruct what the original hole looked like? Such a procedure is routine in autopsies of this sort and should not be considered something out of the ordinary.

In the so-called death certificate that was completed by Rear Admiral George G. Burkley (the physician to the President), the head wound and the back wound were specifically mentioned; the anterior throat wound was not. Why?

The heavily edited official autopsy report was strange in its superficial description of the head damage, which, after all, was the cause of death. Parkland Memorial Hospital surgeons who were physically located near the President in such a way as to see his head wounds clearly reported that there was a wound in the left temple. Such wound was never reported in the autopsy.

The sketch of the top of the President's head made during the autopsy showed a wound in the left forehead; it was indicated as roughly square in outline and over an inch along the side (Fig. 10-1). That wound was ignored in the autopsy report. The fact that the brain was never dissected in accord with long-established practice in such cases and contrary to the directives published for military pathologists made interpretation of the head wounds from the existing record well-nigh impossible.

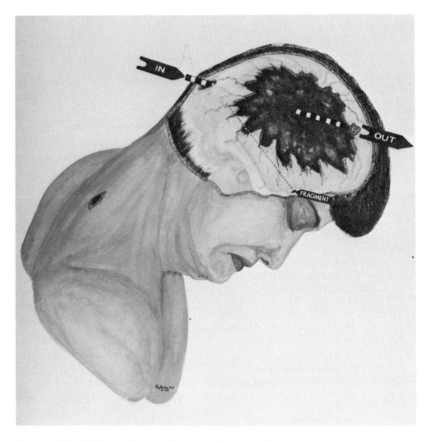

Figure 10-1. This is Warren Commission Exhibit Number 388. It shows an artist's impression of the President's head wound. The drawing was made by a naval enlisted man who never saw the actual wounds nor photographs of the wounds. He drew according to a description given to him by one of the autopsy pathologists who himself had never seen photographs of the head wound. He described what the artist was to draw from unaided memory after months had elapsed. He had no notes or other aids to remembering because (as he certified in writing) he had destroyed all such materials by burning. The extreme flexion of the President's neck at the time of the head shot is not supported by photographs taken moments before the head shot. The inshoot hole does not seem to be in accord with the original autopsy report as to location. The hole as depicted in the back is questionable. Photographs said to be of the late President's back show the hole to be elongated in a lateral not vertical direction; there should be a tailing of the wound in the direction of the right shoulder. As depicted in this sketch, the back wound does not seem to be located at the level of the third thoracic vertebra, the position specified in the death certificate.

The reported loss of the brain by the National Archives plus its previous record of being hidden away strongly suggest that there is information contained in that brain (if the organ has not been willfully destroyed) that would significantly modify the conclusions of the Warren Commission. The reports by FBI agents that "surgery" was done on the President's skull before the Bethesda pathologists began their work have never been clarified.

According to the death certificate, the wound in the back was in the chest region, a statement confirmed by the level of the entrance holes in the President's clothing. In its Report, the Commission managed to call the wound a "neck" wound. A problem still faces the scholar who tries to interpret the wound and to line it up with the anterior throat wound. To do so requires that the shooter had been below the horizontal or might have been at ground level. Any higher elevation would have driven a bullet entering in the back as the Report said it did into the sternum or breastbone.

Doctor Burkley, the rear admiral who was Kennedy's personal physician, apparently edited thoroughly the autopsy report of the pathologists. He also approved the most unusual and professionally questionable destruction of notes by Doctor Humes concerning the autopsy. One might also ask why the late President's personal physician was never asked to testify under oath before the Commission.

The saga of the autopsy illustrations (photographs and x-rays) is beyond belief. The best information to date is that the color photographs were never authenticated; no chain of custody has been revealed; no one can be certain that the photographs being held in the National Archives are, in fact, photographs of the body and the wounds of the deceased President Kennedy. Photographs to establish identity seem never to have been made. The corpse was apparently not fingerprinted.

A Suggestion

Perhaps it would be helpful to rectify in a small way a

critical failure of the Commission. The autopsy pathologists, if they would, and the emergency room surgeons from Parkland Memorial Hospital who treated the President before death, if they would, should be given free access to the complete file of illustrative material so that they could study the material, discuss it among themselves, and over a decade after the event, reconstruct in an orderly fashion just what the dead remains of John F. Kennedy could tell the living about his death. Too much must not be expected from such a meeting. Time has a way of blotting out important details of memory. Nevertheless, there is a bare possibility that some of the inconsistencies and contradictions in the medicolegal aspects of President Kennedy's death could be resolved by such a meeting — assuming that no threatening pressures were exerted on the participants.

The President's Illnesses

Clinch (1973) contends that John F. Kennedy as President was a "very sick man." It is true that during his lifetime, he had assorted illnesses which should have left traces that could have been revealed by an adequate postmortem examination.

A tremor of his hands appeared at various times, notably during a speech given in 1963.

There was evidence that Kennedy suffered repeated bouts of jaundice as a young man. The cause was obscure. He picked up malaria during his service in the Navy in World War II. His back gave him constant pain until the day of his death. The fact of his adrenal insufficiency was well established.

It was strange that no relics of at least some of these pathological conditions were revealed in the microscopic examinations reported to have been made on all pertinent organs of Kennedy's remains.

Was the microscopic examination incompetent or was the report of the examination dishonest?

The cursory and clearly curtailed report of the microscopic study of tissue samples from Kennedy's body throws grave doubts on the competence of the entire autopsy report. If the deficiencies stemmed from "editing" by public officials before publication, those "editors" should be remembered as subversives who helped to destroy faith in the United States and its fundamental legal processes.

The President's Adrenal Pathology

It has been claimed that John F. Kennedy did, in fact, have Addison's disease and was receiving 25 mg cortisone daily plus one 150 mg implant of desoxycorticosterone acetate every three months in 1954 (Clinch, 1973). In 1961, the dosage was said to have been increased. Observers reportedly noted facial edema and other characteristics of cortisone therapy.

Clinch (1973) refers to the study made by L'Etang (1970), who suggests that the exhuberant optimism and careless overconfidence shown by Kennedy may well have been related to his adrenal pathology. The euphoria that accompanies cortisone therapy is alleged to have been indicated by what L'Etang interpreted as defective judgement and inadequate leadership during the crisis of the Bay of Pigs. The later Cuban missile crisis was to bring out brilliant statesmanship by the President. L'Etang interpreted such regular inconsistencies of behavior as being related to Kennedy's adrenal pathology.

Clinch (1973) denies that the admitted adrenal pathology was involved in Kennedy's behavior. She opts for the conclusion that "the fluctuations in his psyche seem to have been more the result of his childhood experiences and his personal and social psychohistory than his medical history." Such psychoanalytic position is valueless and beclouds any attempt to reach a meaningful understanding of John F. Kennedy.

These studies do, however, lend additional support to the author's conclusion that the deletion of data on Kennedy's endocrine system, as a result of gross and microscopic examination of the several endocrine organs, proves that critical pathology was found and the evidence was suppressed.

Who Was Involved?

From a study of the medicolegal aspects of the J.F. Kennedy

murder, it is of course not possible to point out specific persons or agencies who might have had a direct connection with the death. There are, however, matters of record that suggest directions one might take in an attempt to trace such relations.

A comment made by Prouty (1973) in his book on what he calls the "secret team" is suggestive. "Whether or not the Secret Team had anything whatsoever to do with the deaths of Rafael Trujillo, Ngo Dinh Diem, Ngo Dinh Nhu, Dag Hammerskjold, John F. Kennedy, Robert F. Kennedy, Martin Luther King, and others may never be revealed, but what is known is that the power of the Team is enchanced by the 'cult of the gun' . . ."

Prouty comments on the CIA and its relations with the late President Kennedy and the peculiar relation between the secret team and President Johnson that may be implied as a result of the assassination. "In the face of these shocking events, who could have expected a man who had been in the range of gunfire that ended the life of his predecessor, to make any moves in those critical days that would indicate he was not going to go along with the pressures which had surfaced so violently in Dallas? He knew exactly what had happened there in Dallas. He did not need to wait for the further findings of the Warren Commission. He already knew that the death of Lee Harvey Oswald would never bring any relief to him or his successors" (Prouty, 1973, p. 416).*

Which Autopsy Report?

Commission Exhibit Number 387 was the autopsy report as

---

*On 18 May 1964 John A. McCone, as Director of The Central Intelligence Agency, swore that Lee Harvey Oswald was never in any capacity at any time employed by the CIA, that the CIA never had contact with him nor attempted to have such at any time for any purpose, that in no manner or form did the CIA furnish him with any funds at any time directly or indirectly, and that Oswald was never directly or indirectly in any manner whatsoever associated or connected with the CIA at any time. A copy of this strongly worded affadavit was published on page 866, volume 17 of the Hearings of the Warren Commission as Commission Exhibit Number 870. The document left no room for future "clarification." If current rumors and developments with respect to CIA relationships to the Kennedy murder become firm, a serious question of official perjury and deceit faces the nation.

it reached the public. *It was not dated.* That lack has never been explained. Preliminary drafts, notes, and other papers connected directly to the autopsy findings were destroyed by Doctor Humes, the pathologist in charge of the autopsy. Precisely what papers were destroyed is not known.

The introductory section of the autopsy report as published contained gratuitous statements about the number of shots fired and from where they came. At the time the report was written, these "facts" were not yet established; they were yet to be sifted by the Commission. The writer or writers of the published version of the autopsy report included as demonstrated fact matters that were still under investigation. Or were they?

The dearth of factual data collected from the emergency room personnel at Parkland Memorial Hospital raises the question of why? The official military *Autopsy Manual* directs that adequate clinical data be abstracted in the introductory part of the protocol. Failure of the pathologists to consult with surgeons in Dallas who had treated Kennedy, *before* they initiated anatomical dissection was contrary to accepted standards of professional practice and not in accord with military directives. It is indeed difficult to explain or justify the oversight.

Internally the autopsy report was inadequate. Attempts by responsible officials of the American Medical Association to obtain clarification of serious omissions have been ignored by government officials, including top-level medical officers in the Navy.

A grave internal defect of the autopsy report was the lack of any reference to the adrenal glands. Such information would not explain the death of the President, but it is requested in military directives covering the conduct of an adequate autopsy. Lack of such information demonstrates questionable understanding on the part of the pathologists of what ought to have been included in the autopsy of the victim in a case of international significance or a deliberate deletion of information for political reasons.

In the November 1965 issue of *Current Medicine for*

Attorneys, it was pointed out that "the question is, was President Kennedy 'impaired for public life' when he ran for office — by reason of adrenal pathology. Certainly the absence of findings in the autopsy on this point suggest that he was" (1965).

A censored, edited, mutilated, and possibly fictionalized autopsy report is not authoritative. Moreover, it can but poorly serve to reconstruct the murder scenario of John F. Kennedy.

The crime involved is not merely one of political cover-up for whatever reason; it is not the giving of aid, comfort, and protection to a presidential murderer or murderers. The crime is more vicious than that; it is an evil spewed out on mankind; it is a deliberate distortion of history that cannot be justified or explained away. The perpetrators have done their work well; they have raped truth; they have sown and fertilized distrust of government. In the process they have dehumanized themselves and will forever see branded on their souls the mark of the traitor, the defiler of all that is good in *Homo sapiens.*

Newcomb and Adams (1974) have proposed an explanation of the John F. Kennedy assassination that involves a small number of government officials and Secret Service agents. Selected members of the latter group are held to have murdered him. It is further postulated that the plan was well worked out and left no possibility of President Kennedy's leaving the motorcade alive. The medicolegal evidence itself neither supports nor denies this view.

The case can be made for murder of John F. Kennedy by members of the central government. According to the author, however, some of the interpretations and assumptions that go with it are more difficult to accept than is the official version of the murder.

The difficulty with the theory of an assassin being part of the official party is that no disinterested witness can be found who even hints that such an "inside job" was observed.

The fact that more than one person was involved in the killing seems more probable than the lone, lonesome killer proposed by the Warren Commission.

An exasperating aspect of the entire affair was the strange manner in which the Secret Service conducted itself before, during, and after the event. This strange behavior has been aped by other central government agencies, including officials of the National Archives. Secrecy that seems to have no apparent need or justification does not engender confidence in a public agency. Such secrecy has turned many thoughtful scholars against the National Archives officials and others in key government positions. If there are no secrets, why the bullheaded refusal to permit adequate study of the case files of the J.F. Kennedy murder *in toto?* If there are secrets, the light of day would perhaps kill some of the mold of distrust, cynicism, and disaffection seen by many honest citizens as spreading over the entire central government machine.

Handling of Evidence

The total evidence connected with the murder of John F. Kennedy was handled in an unconventional manner; the result was clearly damaging to the solution of the case. The Secret Service received the following materials relevant to the murder: films and x-rays taken at autopsy; various versions of the autopsy report; the President's limousine and the windshield damaged by a bullet fragment; presumably all the clothing of John F. Kennedy; three pieces of Kennedy's skull; key assassination witnesses; two bullets allegedly part of the murder action; photos of the event; recordings of Dallas Police Department radio traffic; television and radio recordings of press interviews with doctors from Parkland Memorial Hospital; first reconstruction of the event; and interviews with Oswald's wife.

Of this mass of evidence only the following was shared with the FBI: autopsy report; windshield from the presidential limousine; Kennedy's clothing; the two bullets; photos of the event; witnesses; police radio recordings; and interview data of Marina Oswald.

The Warren Commission received only these: the autopsy report, windshield, clothing (at least part), bullets, photos of the event, witnesses, police radio log, and Marina Oswald interviews.

It is of interest that all the evidence received by the FBI was given to the Warren Commission. Crucial evidence in the hands of the Secret Service was kept from the Warren Commission; some of that evidence has been "classified," lost, strayed, or misplaced while presumably part of the National Archives holdings.

The Pathologists and the Single Bullet

An interesting exchange took place between Representative Ford and Colonel Finck with respect to the unanimous conclusions of the autopsy team. On page 383 of volume 2 in the Commission Hearings, Representative Ford said, "I believe you testified, Colonel, that you concurred on the previous testimony of Commander Humes and Commander Boswell, and that you are one of the co-authors of the autopsy. At any time during this process where you were conducting the autopsy, was there any disagreement between any one of you three, any difference of opinion as to anything involved in the autopsy?" Colonel Finck answered curtly, "No, sir." Representative Ford pursued this line, presumably so that there would be no question whatever about the answer. He said, "There has been complete unanimity on what you saw, what you did, and what you reported?" Colonel Finck again answered, "Yes, sir." Colonel Finck, under oath, testified that there was complete agreement on the matter of the autopsy observations and conclusions.

The agreement has implications for the mysterious bullet which presumably went through President Kennedy, smashed a rib in Governor Connally, and smashed Governor Connally's wrist. Commander Humes stated clearly in his testimony that the pristine bullet, showing no deformation or loss of particles, could not have caused the wrist wound in Governor Connally. Colonel Finck confirmed that the bullet in question could not have caused the severe damage to Governor Connally's wrist.

This contention about the pristine bullet, according to

Colonel Finck's responses to Representative Ford, was a conclusion agreed upon unanimously by the autopsy team. Therefore, in the face of a strong, unanimous, professional opinion based upon observations by qualified pathologists, it would seem imperative that these observations and conclusions be made part of any conclusion that the Commission were to arrive at.

In the light of the strength and weight of the pathologists' testimony concerning the mysterious undeformed bullet, it was unacceptable for the Commission to conclude that the bullet did in fact smash the rib and wrist of Governor Connally.* There was a problem in that the conclusion by the Commission was completely out of line with and unsupported by the testimony, observations, and interpretations of the autopsy team. The Commission apparently did not understand what it was doing; or, for some reason not apparent in the twenty-six volumes of the Hearings, it saw fit to create a fictional situation, i.e. the single bullet going through the upper part of President Kennedy's body, making a virtually right-angle turn in midair, then passing through Governor Connally's body causing severe bone damage, and ending up in the Governor's thigh in an undeformed, unmutilated condition. This theory has never been satisfactorily explained either by the Commission Report or by the subsequent apologists for the Commission Report.

The author is not suggesting that the Commission members were knaves, crooks, liars, or evil men. There are no available data upon which to build such a theory. However, when taken altogether, the scientific data inescapably forces a denial of the

---

*On 21 April 1964 a conference was held to decide just when the first and second bullets hit as compared to the Zapruder film frames. Present at the conference was Doctor F. W. Light, Jr., probably one of the most knowledgeable experimental pathologists in the field of wound ballistics; Doctor Joseph Dolce, a respected consultant in wound ballistics to Edgewood Arsenal, was also present. After the formal showing of the Zapruder film there was a discussion. "In a discussion after the conference Drs. Light and Dolce expressed themselves as being very strongly of the opinion that Connally had been hit by two different bullets, principally on the grounds that the bullet removed from Connally's stretcher could not have broken his radius without having suffered more distortion" (Eisenberg, 1964).

validity of the single bullet idea with respect to the nonfatal wound in Kennedy and the devastating bone damage in Governor Connally. Further than that, no conclusions can be formulated until the complete scientific autopsy data and materials are available for objective examination by scientists who are experts in forensic biology and forensic pathology. Until a free, uncluttered, and uncontrolled examination of what materials still exist is made, there is an area of uncertainty, an area which leaves open more questions than were allegedly answered by the conclusions of the Presidential Commission taking evidence in the murder of President Kennedy.

The single bullet theory was constructed out of whole cloth. It is a published lie arrived at only by ignoring the unanimous conclusions of the three pathologists who performed the autopsy on Kennedy's remains.

Some Conclusions

The discrepancies and confusing aspects of the medicolegal investigation of President Kennedy's murder are many and complex. Perhaps some are understandable errors; others clearly are planned diversionary efforts.* A recapitulation of some items of concern may be useful in understanding why so many forensic scientists have been dissatisfied with the results of the Warren Commission's deliberations.

- Parkland Memorial Hospital surgeons who attended the stricken President observed a small, round wound in the anterior neck of the President, which they interpreted as a bullet entrance hole. No other forensic science experts saw that wound.
- Interpretation of the fatal head wound by several attending

---

*Wrone (1972) is unequivocal as a historian about his conclusions concerning the murder of President Kennedy. He contends that public documents demonstrate the existence of a conspiracy; no evidence having probative value links Oswald to the specific act of firing at Kennedy; the evidence as it exists does not tie into the murder, the official military establishment, American business, governmental spying agencies of the United States, France, or Russia, or left wing groups. The evaluations made in this book are in accord with Wrone's conclusions.

surgeons suggested a high-velocity handgun bullet fired at close range.

- Attending surgeons who rendered aid to the moribund President observed and described a gunshot wound in the left temple. This wound was later ignored by the investigating Commission.

- The dead President's remains were spirited away illegally out of the jurisdiction of the Dallas coroner by the use of force, violence, and subterfuge on the part of federal officials. Texas law prohibits removal of a body from the state without an autopsy.

- Governor Connally's wounds were clearly caused by a separate bullet that passed through his body at an angle of about 25 degrees downward. The clothing he wore at the time of the shooting was cleaned and pressed before laboratory tests could be carried out on it. This crucial evidence was destroyed. Some of the holes in the clothing were also modified in size and shape so that the FBI laboratory technicians could conclude very little about them.

- An inadequate autopsy was performed on the President's remains at Bethesda Naval Hospital. Critical directions spelled out in the official Armed Forces Institute of Pathology *Autopsy Manual* were flagrantly ignored by the military autopsy pathologists, probably under orders from superior officers.

- A mysterious bullet of unverified origin and in questionable condition was used by the Warren Commission as serious and indeed key evidence.

- The head wounds as described by the pathologists at Bethesda seemed to be different than the head wound described by the attending surgeons. According to FBI agents O'Neill and Sibert, who were present at the autopsy, "surgery" had been performed in the head area of the corpse some time before it was unwrapped at Bethesda. This report has never been clarified.

- The autopsy pathologists never knew about the anterior neck wound as it was before the tracheotomy incision until the day after the autopsy was completed.

- According to Agent Kellerman, the President exhibited no facial injuries while at Parkland Memorial Hospital. Apparently the face was disfigured when seen by the Bethesda pathologists and later by the family, even after the mortician's cosmetician had performed his service.
- Microscopic sections of the neck wound tissue showed "foreign substances such as fibre particles" in the wound, a condition characteristic of an entrance, not an exit wound.
- Odd pieces of skull, presumably from the President's head, were brought to the pathologists by Secret Service Agents when the autopsy was nearly over. Other fragments appeared and disappeared during the days after the autopsy.
- Position of the alleged entrance hole in the posterior region of the skull was described at one point by the autopsy pathologists and at another point 4 inches higher by a panel that reviewed the photographs (said to have been made at the autopsy) in 1968.
- Most, if not all, of the photographs said to have been taken at the autopsy are unverified and may have no probative value.

All these items are matters of substance. They deserve serious consideration in any reevaluation of the entire Warren Commission Report. At the present, however, the weight of these questions is such as to vitiate the conclusions published by the Warren Commission.

A SUMMATION

In discussing the mysteries of the John F. Kennedy assassination, Miss Cooper (1973) develops an interesting summary of the murder. She relies heavily on the work of Doctor Cyril Wecht, who at the present time is Coroner of Allegheny County in Pennsylvania. The official conclusion of the Warren Commission was to the effect that Kennedy was shot from the rear by an individual named Lee Harvey Oswald. Oswald was said to have been standing at a window on the sixth floor of a building known as the Texas School Book Depository. The

Commission concluded that Oswald acted alone and that there was no conspiracy of any kind involved in the murder. The Commission also maintained that three shots and three shots only were fired. They concluded that the first shot went into President Kennedy's back and out his throat. Then in some way that bullet was said to have made a turn in the air and wounded Governor Connally on the extreme right side. The second bullet was said to have entered the President's brain, destroying it and a good portion of his skull and killing him instantly. The third shot has never been accounted for. It is classified as a mystery.

The various arguments and theories with respect to what actually happened are secondary to the most critical question, which involved where the bullets did, in fact, enter the President's body, how many bullets actually were fired, and where any of these bullets exited. In other words, the key question is connected to physical evidence that can show where the bullets came from, where they struck the President, and what organs and tissues were actually destroyed in the process. A bullet entrance hole is usually not too difficult to identify. It is ordinarily round. It is somewhat smaller than the diameter of the bullet because the skin tends to contract after the bullet passes through it. The exit hole is usually larger than the entrance hole because the bullet may be tumbling and tends to rip and tear tissue and push it away in front of it.

Three physicians in the military service were called upon to perform the autopsy on President Kennedy. These physicians were Commander James J. Humes, Commander J. Thornton Boswell, both of the Navy Medical Corps, and Lieutenant Colonel Pierre Finck, who was in the Army Medical Corps. None of these physicians had practical firsthand experience with bullet wounds. The Navy doctors were hospital pathologists who collectively, apparently, had only one case of gunshot wounds to their credit. Doctor Finck was what one might call an administrative pathologist who reviewed other cases and published material that was in the files of the Armed Forces Institute of Pathology. His experience with gunshot wounds at the autopsy table was extremely limited. From the very beginning of this entire investigation, difficulties arose. The highly skilled surgeons in Parkland Hospital in Dallas, Texas, first saw the wound in the President's throat just below the larynx. They described it as being about 3 to 5 mm in diameter or about 1/5 of an inch. This was an extremely small hole. It is compatible with the entrance hole of a bullet, and indeed, several of the surgeons referred to that wound in the front of the throat as an entrance hole. The doctors who performed the autopsy described the wound in Kennedy's back as being from 4 to 7 mm in diameter. This was obviously a larger wound than the one in the anterior part of the neck. It is a proper question to ask in this case why the alleged entrance wound was larger than the exit wound. Such a situation may occur, but it is usually seen in contact wounds of the skull and not in distant wounds through soft tissue.

Doctor Wecht has suggested that there is a good possibility that the late President's wound in the anterior part of the neck was really an entrance wound as several of the surgeons said. Moreover, he suggested that the back wound, which he examined only through photographs, had some characteristics of a gunshot wound.

There was further confusion concerning the location of the wound in the President's back. It changed position with different versions of the autopsy report. The chart done at the autopsy showed the wound in the back as being about 4 to 6 inches below the neck. In one version of the autopsy, the pathologists said that the wound was at the nape of the neck. The holes in the President's suit coat and shirt indicated clearly that these holes were 6 inches below the top of the collar. Where then was the hole in the President's back? It has been suggested that the President was raising his arms to wave to the crowd, hiking up his shirt and jacket so that the holes there lined up with a real hole in the nape of his neck. However, the photographs made at the time the shot occurred indicates that the President did not have his hands up in the air, but he was sitting in a relaxed position with his arm on the arm rest of the automobile.

It is difficult to figure out how the bullet entered 4 inches below the neck in the back and exited slightly below the larynx or Adam's apple in the front of the throat. This would have required an upward course of the bullet through the President's body. One suggestion was that the bullet hit something in the body and ricocheted upward. However, this was denied by the Warren Commission and by x-rays, which indicate that no bone or hard tissue of any sort was struck by this bullet. One cannot argue either that the President was leaning forward causing the bullet to take this track. At the time of the shooting, the President could not lean forward because he was wearing a canvas brace with metal stays in it, which was wrapped with an Ace bandage. In this rigid frame he had to sit upright.

Of greater difficulty, of course, is the single bullet theory proposed by the Warren Commission. This theory maintains that the bullet entered the President's back and went out through the front of his throat, then made a right-angle turn in midair, went into Governor Connally's body in the extreme right of his back, tearing out a portion of his fifth rib. From there it went on downward, smashing his right wrist, which happened to be resting on his left thigh, and entered his thigh, leaving a chunk of metal in the thigh bone. The bullet was said to have fallen out of the wound in his thigh. It is true that bullets do some strange things and describe weird patterns in body tissues. However, in the air, there is not this kind of erratic behavior; bullets follow the normal laws of physics that govern all flying objects. Governor Connally had time to turn around when he heard the first shot and maintained, as did his wife, that it was "inconceivable" that he was struck with the same bullet that hit Kennedy.

The bullet said to have done all this damage on two individuals probably weighed somewhere between 160 and 161 grains before it was fired. After allegedly penetrating seven layers of skin plus two large bones, it weighed 159 grains. If true, this is a modern miracle, for most bullets are deformed when they strike bone and, in the process, lose significant amounts of metal. In addition, metal particles were seen in x-rays taken of Governor Connally's wrist and thigh, and there were metal particles allegedly left in the President's body. If this bullet were pristine, undeformed, and had lost very little weight, it is not in keeping with the laws of physics that it could have caused all the harm it was said to have caused.

An important aspect of the examination of the fatal wound to the President's head would have been an examination of the brain itself, which was preserved in formaldehyde. Bullets, when they go through brain tissue, leave a track; generally the brain is hardened in formaldehyde and then very carefully dissected in order to follow the path that the bullet or bullet fragments may have taken. According to records in the National Archives, the brain of the President was in existence a year and one-half after Kennedy was murdered. At that time, Admiral Burkley, transferring various materials to the National Archives, listed in a memorandum various autopsy materials including the brain and microscopic slides made at the autopsy. Admiral Burkley was Kennedy's personal physician. Strangely enough, the brain and the slides have disappeared. Where they are, nobody admits to knowing. Despite the fact that the slides and the brain have disappeared, there are some large photographs of the late President's brain. In the front part of the right cerebral hemisphere of the brain in one of the photographs available, there was a dark brownish black object that had a white glistening effect. It measured about 13 by 20 mm or about 3/4 by 1 1/2 inches. The object could have been larger than it appeared in the photograph because brain material around it hid the borders of this object. This unidentified object was at no time mentioned in the final autopsy report produced by the military pathologists. Despite the fact that some thirty-five pieces of metal, some no bigger than a grain of sand, were accounted for from the bullet in the President's head, this larger object was ignored.

What was this object? It could have been the remains of a hemorrhage caused by the gunshot wounds. It could have been a piece of metal or a respectable chunk of a bullet fragment. Finally, it could have been a brain tumor or some kind of a malformation in the blood vessels in that part of the brain. It seems proper to exclude a hemorrhage caused by a gunshot wound. If such a hemorrhage existed, it is inconceivable that pathologists who performed the autopsy would not have recorded it. Because of its size, one can hardly accept that the three doctors who performed the autopsy did not see it. The only conclusion one can come to is that this particular object, whatever it might have been, was purposely and willfully omitted from the report. For what reason, of course, one cannot, on the basis of the evidence, make any statement.

Supposing that the object was a bullet or a fragment of a bullet, where did this bullet come from or where did the fragment come from? Is there an indication that there was another gunman and that Kennedy received two shots to the head instead of one?

There was another odd aspect to the autopsy according to an examination of the autopsy photographs. These photographs showed a loose flap of skin on the left side of the back part of the late President's head. Careful examination of the entire twenty-six volumes of the Warren Commission Report failed to reveal anywhere that this wound was mentioned. It certainly was not mentioned in the autopsy report. However, when the twenty-six volumes of the Warren Commission Report were reexamined, there was a brief word from Doctor Marion Jenkins, who referred to this wound when Kennedy was brought into Parkland Hospital. According to Doctor Jenkins, this wound was bleeding, a fact that demonstrates that it was made before death, and that in all probability it was related to the shooting incident. In other words, it was not the result of careless handling of the President's body during transportation after death. Doctor Wecht, who has examined this photograph, contended that the wound was too small to have resulted from the passage of the whole bullet, but in all probability resulted from a fragment of a bullet passing out through the flap.

This flaplike wound is more important than meets the eye, for if the President were shot in the back with a bullet that traveled through his throat, and if he were also shot in the head by a bullet coming from the right and the rear as the Warren Commission contended, it would be difficult to look at a wound on the left side of the head without a certain amount of suspicion. It is incomprehensible that this wound was not examined at the autopsy and described thoroughly. In fact, there is really no evidence from the autopsy that the pathologists did a thorough search of the President's head to see whether more than one bullet hit him in the head. As far as is known, the hair was not combed carefully to identify other entrance wounds. Usually, when there is a question of bullet wounds to the head that might be hidden, the hair is combed and even parts of this hair are shaved off to get a clearer picture of what occurred. The mysteriously missing brain might give some information about this odd wound on the left side of the rear of the late President's skull.

The administrative nonsense associated with these materials is beyond belief. Various panels were called together to examine the evidence. For example, Attorney General Ramsey Clark called together a number of pathologists to reexamine the assassination materials. They came up with the proper answer to satisfy governmental sources. The first medical man who was permitted to see these materials as an individual was not a forensic scientist, was not a pathologist, was not an expert in crime detection, but was a urologist.

The written record of the autopsy certainly suggests that the pathologists involved did a dismal job. However, one must realize that they were military officers on active duty, and the charitable view is to submit that they were not allowed to reveal all the facts they found. It is a safe contention to claim that their report was changed at some later date. It also seems evident that during the actual autopsy, they were under some kind of unethical control, probably by the Secret Service or the military. This suggestion has merit when one examines the sworn testimony Doctor Finck made at the trial of Clay Shaw in New Orleans. Doctor Finck was asked why the pathologists did not carry out the routine, standard, ordinary task of dissecting the wound in President Kennedy's back. This dissection would have revealed the path of the bullet. Doctor Finck swore under oath that the pathologists were told not to dissect that wound. How such a mistake could come about is hard to understand. The fact remains it did come about.

The complete autopsy report as written by the pathologists

was altered during its route through military channels. Certain sections were removed. Admiral George Burkley, who was President Kennedy's personal physician, admitted that he doctored the autopsy report. What happened to the first report that went to Admiral Burkley? Two months passed before he released portions of the autopsy. Probably the other parts were destroyed in some way. This is not a frivolous suggestion because the first report that was written, the original draft that indicated where the bullets went into the body and came out of the body; the report that indicated where the wounds were, how many bullets were there, and the paths of these bullets; the report that indicated whether any bullets were still in Kennedy's body, was burned by Doctor Humes, who wrote it. It is very difficult to understand how the original draft of such an important autopsy could be burned.

One wonders also about the peculiarity of certain missing facts. For example, it is known that the pathologists actually examined President Kennedy's adrenal glands. Doctor Boswell, one of the pathologists at the autopsy, admitted that the adrenal glands were identified. Were they diseased? It must be concluded firmly that they were diseased and probably showed that the late President suffered from Addison's disease. If they had not been diseased, then the doctors and the politicians would have been happy to discuss these healthy adrenal glands at great length in order to end any rumors. Could it have been that the large object seen in the photograph of the President's brain was, in fact, a tumor (either benign or malignant) that was the root cause of his adrenal problems?

Paulette Cooper concludes her evaluation of the Warren Commission Report with this paragraph. "But these are speculations which may never be satisfied because the parts of the body that could prove or disprove them — the brain — is missing together with vital portions of the autopsy report. Withholding or altering information has fostered exactly what the public and the government would have preferred ended: rumors, series, and insinuations of conspiracy."

It is ironic that presumably sophisticated government bureaucrats and politicians did not understand one of the elementary facts of living: A lie begets further lies. A simple, possibly harmless, series of lies incorporated in the Warren Commission Report required further lies to cover up the original lies. A chain reaction of one lie is then built upon another continuously in order to cover the track of prevarication. The average citizen understands this. How government bureaucrats were unaware of this fact suggests something is wrong with our choosing of governmental leaders. Something is wrong with our system of education that permits individuals of this sort to rise to high levels of public responsibility without a keen awareness of the devastating results of lying as official policy. To argue that the end result was so important that it justified these lies is reprehensible, naive, and counterproductive. No lie can ever be justified in terms of the end result. For, in the long run, an official lie begins a chain of further lies, so that when the truth finally surfaces, there is revealed a stinking morass of interlocking lies that cause long-term, if not permanent, damage to the government subscribing to such a procedure.

AUTOPSY PROCEDURE

As the first part of this Appendix, detailed directions for conducting any autopsy are taken verbatim from the official *Autopsy Manual* written by the staff of the prestigious Armed Forces Institute of Pathology and adopted by the three military services as a directive. Illustrations from the original have been deleted because they are not all directly pertinent to the discussion in this book.

The second part of this Appendix reprints a medical article that reflects current professional standards for medicolegal investigations of death.

TECHNIQUE OF THE AUTOPSY

Section I. INSTRUCTIONS

Preparatory Measures

a. Before he performs the autopsy, the pathologist should familiarize himself with the clinical history, clinical diagnosis, and special points of interest to the clinician. Direct consultation with the responsible clinician is desirable. A complete review of the patient's hospital records will furnish valuable information and may indicate special procedures which otherwise might not be carried out.

b. The final typed autopsy protocol must include a clinical abstract for reviewing pathologists who do not have access to the clinical records.

c. The prosector should be familiar with chapter 6 in the case of medicolegal autopsies and Armed Forces Directives in appendix I. The body must be identified. The prosector must assure himself that the autopsy is authorized.

d. During the autopsy the prosector will ligate all major blood vessels in a manner that will permit recovery of the vessles during the embalming. It is desired that the ligatures be of sufficient length and firmly tied to facilitate recovery. The degree of consideration given by the prosector will have a strong influence on the eventual quality of preservation and appearance of the body.

Inspection

a. Both the anterior and posterior surfaces should be scrutinized. The more important observations include signs of violence, fractures, recent or healed wounds and lacerations, identifying marks, such as tattoos, edema of the legs, back, scrotum, or face, distention of the abdomen, jaundice, hemorrhage from the orifices of the body, hemorrhage into the subcutaneous tissues or cornea, decubital ulcers, abnormal pigmentation, tumors, anomalies, deformities, distribution of hair and subcutaneous fat, and symmetry of the trunk and extremities. The oral and nasal cavities should be examined and the state of the mucosa noted. The number, character, and state of preservation of the teeth may be indicative of certain lesions or diseases. The eyelids should be elevated and the color, size, and shape of both pupils recorded, with other pertinent observations. The external genitalia should be examined.

b. If the patient has received radioactive material, precautions are indicated in paragraphs 105 and 106.

Primary Incision of Thorax and Abdomen

a. The usual incision for both men and women is the **Y**-shaped incision . . . This begins at a point near the acromial extremity of the clavicle, extends in a curve below the corresponding breast to the xyphiod process of the sternum, and thence in similar manner to the opposite acromial extremity. From the xyphoid process, the incision is extended downward in the midline to the symphysis pubis, passing to the left of the umbilicus and not entering the peritoneum.

b. When the autopsy permit restricts examination of the thorax or abdomen, the skin incisions should be modified to allow individual exposure of either of these cavities without cutting into the skin of the adjacent restricted area. Transforming the lower end of the abdominal incision into an inverted **V** allows easier dissection of the inguinal region and the femoral triangle. An extension of the primary incisions down the anteromedial aspect of the arm may be made . . . However, special permission is required.

c. The peritoneum is incised with scissors, or with a knife placed between two of the prosector's fingers as guides to avoid injury to the intestines or other viscera. The attachments of the abdominal wall to the costal border are severed to lay open the abdominal cavity. Transverse incisions of the rectus muscles are made when necessary to permit easier access to the peritoneal cavity. The incision over the thorax should extend through the skin, subcutaneous fat, and muscle, so that these tissues can be dissected away from the bony thoracic wall as far superiorly as 2 cm. above the sternoclavicular joints.

Skin

Random ellipses of skin, 2 to 3 cm. in length, may be obtained adjacent to the primary incision. Lesions noted in the external examination may be removed by excising a small ellipse which includes the subcutaneous tissue as well as the dermis. The *skin of the face, neck, arms, and hands must not be incised except when specific permission is granted.* If more than one lesion is removed, each should be placed in a separate bottle and the site of origin indicated on the label.

Inspection of the Peritoneal Cavity and Abdominal Organs

The amount of fluid, the character of the surfaces, and the presence of adhesions should be noted. The size, character, and position of the omentum may yield information concerning focal lesions within the abdomen. The size and relative position of each of the viscera should be observed in relation to fixed landmarks; for example, the liver might be noted as extending so many centimeters below the right and left costal margins in the mid-clavicular lines.

Fluid in Peritoneal Cavity

Cultures and smears should be obtained if indicated. When the amount of fluid in the cavity is increased, save at least 50 cc. in a clean dry vessel. If warranted, determine the specific gravity and the character of the cells in the centrifugal sediment.

Exposure and Inspection of the Thoracic Viscera

a. If pneumothorax is suspected, insert a 16 gauge needle, attached to a 25 cc. syringe filled with water, through an intercostal space into the pleural cavity. Bubbles will appear in the syringe if there is air under pressure.

b. Open the thorax by cutting the costal cartilages just medial to the costochondral junction. The knife should always be directed away from the subject's face to avoide possible damage. Use a heavy cartilage knife for this purpose, with the edge of the blade parallel to the surface of the body to prevent the point from entering the pleural cavity and puncturing a lung. If the cartilages are calcified, rib shears or a saw must be used. Disarticulate the sternoclavicular joints by cutting the capsular ligaments. Sever the first rib with rib shears. Dissect the diaphragm free from the lower ribs on both sides, and remove the triangular "chest plate" to expose the heart, superior mediastinum, and pleural cavities. It is advisable to place a hemostat on the internal mammary arteries and veins on each side as they turn from the sternum to enter the superior mediastinum. This will prevent the leadage of blood into the pleural cavities before they have been inspected.

Pleural Cavities

a. The pleural cavities should be inspected before they are contaminated by the prosector's hands. If indicated by the appearance of the fluid or by the history, take samples for culture. When there is appreciable fluid, save 50 cc. in a clean vessel and determine its specific gravity if necessary. The cells can be studied by making smears of the sediment.

b. If there are slight fibrous adhesions, they may be freed by blunt dissection, but if the adhesions are dense it may be necessary to cut around the diaphragm and separate the parietal pleura from the underlying intercostal muscles and ribs in order to remove the lung. If dense adhesions are broken by force, the adjacent lung tissue is often torn.

Thoracic Duct

The prosector should develop the habit of displaying the thoracic duct routinely. It is difficult to demonstrate and must be located before other dissections in the thorax are carried out. Lift the entire right lung from its cavity and draw it to the left side of the body, anterior to the left thoracic cage. This maneuver exposes the right side of the posterior mediastinum. The thoracic duct is located between the aorta and the azygos vein, close to the vertebrae. Opposite the fifth thoracic vertebrae the duct inclines toward the left side and enters the superior mediastinal cavity. It ends by opening into the angle of junction of the left subclavian vein with the left internal jugular vein. The thoracic duct is most easily found just above the diaphragm, to the right and behind the aorta. It can be traced inferiorly below the diaphragm where it joins the cisterna chyli located in front of the second lumbar vertebra.

Pericardial Cavity

The pericardial cavity is opened by a linear incision from below, cutting to the base. Note the amount of fluid, the condition of the surfaces, and the presence of adhesions. A specimen of the heart's blood may be taken for culture if indicated.

Superior Mediastinum

Do this dissection after removal of the heart and lungs so that the pericardial and pleural cavities will not be obscured by blood, or divide the left innominate vein between ligatures as it crosses high in the superior mediastinum, so that the three major branches of the arch of the aorta can be fully visualized. Ligate these branches as close to the parent vessel as feasible. The ligatures should be at least 15 inches long after they are tied. The vessels are now severed below the ligatures and the long strings left attached as an aid to the embalmer in locating the vessels. The thymus or its remnants should be dissected from the tissues of the superior mediastinum, weighed, measured, and examined. Fix all or part of the thymus for microscopic study.

Section II. GENERAL PRINCIPLES IN DISSECTION AND EXAMINATION OF THE VISCERA

General Considerations

a. The following general considerations should be borne in mind in the dissection of the viscera:

(1) The primary incisions in each organ should be so placed as to —

(*a*) Expose the largest possible surface.

(*b*) Open the structures that enter through the hilum.

(*c*) Make visible the ductal and vascular systems.

(*d*) Preserve the orientation and relations of the organ.

(2) All further incisions should, as far as possible, parallel the first.

b. No organ should be separated from a connecting structure until the intervening tissue has been dissected and examined; for example, the ostia of the renal arteries, the renal arteries and veins, and the ureters should be examined before the kidneys are removed from the body; the ampulla, the bile ducts, the gallbladder, the portal vein and the hepatic artery should be examined before the liver is separated from the stomach and the duodenum; and the mesentery, mesenteric arteries and veins should be explored before the intestine is separated from the mesentery.

c. All viscera except the heart should be weighed and measured before they are sectioned. Blood is lost from the cut surface and the weight may be reduced as much as 20 percent. In general the weight, the greatest length, breadth and depth should be recorded. In some organs special measurements are indicated; for example, the circumference of the heart valve rings, the thickness of the walls of the heart, of the cortex and of the combined cortex and medulla of each kidney . . .

d. The blocks to be selected for histological study are indicated under the separate organs. In all cases the prosector should use his judgment in the removal of additional blocks to illustrate specific lesions.

e. All calculi should be saved in a clean dry vessel for subsequent chemical analysis, if indicated.

Removal of Viscera

Two general methods are available, each of which must be modified to meet special situations and the preferences of the prosector. These are: "Organ by Organ Removal" and "Removal of the Viscera En Masse." A third method, "Removal by Systems" is a compromise between the two. It is not described in this manual though it has many advantages and is used by many pathologists.

Section III. ORGAN BY ORGAN REMOVAL

Heart

a. Inspect and palpate the heart *in situ.* Make a longitudinal incision in the pulmonary artery and examine for emboli. Elevate the apex of the heart and sever the inferior vena cava, and the pulmonary veins at their pericardial reflection. Place traction directed inferiorly on the heart and sever the superior vena cava, the aortic valve and the pulmonary artery. Remove the heart from the pericardial sac. Sever the previously opened pulmonary artery 2 cm. above the pulmonary valve. Dissect the proximal portion of the pulmonary artery from the underlying root of the aorta; this allows the aortic valve to be opened later without cutting through the pulmonary artery. Open the coronary arteries by a series of transverse incisions spaced about 2 mm. apart.

b. The preferred method of opening the heart is to follow the blood flow. Dissect the heart as follows: Insert an amputation knife or scissors in the opening of the inferior vena cava and cut through to the opening of the superior vena cava. Use of the grooved director is helpful in making this incision. Open the right auricular appendage with an oblique incision beginning at the center of the previous incision. Cut through the right lateral border of the heart by directing the knife through the tricuspid valve.

c. Open the outflow tract of the right ventricle by cutting the wall of the right ventricle parallel to and about 1 cm. away from the ventricular septum, passing through the valve at the junction of the anterior cusps, continuing the incision to connect with the previous incision in the pulmonary artery.

d. Open the left atrium by cutting between the openings of the pulmonary veins and making another incision from the opening of the left pulmonary vein to the tip of the left auricular appendage. Open the left ventricle by inserting the amputation knife through the opening of the mitral valve and stabbing it through the wall of the left ventricle in the region of the apex, and incise the ventricle along its lateral border, directing the knife through the valve near the lateral junction of the aortic leaflet and posterior leaflet of the mitral valve. The left ventricular cavity can now be partially opened and any blood clots removed. Exend the incision to the apex of the heart.

e. Open the left ventricular outflow tract by directing the amputation knife up through the aortic leaflet of the mitral valve. Make the incision lateral to the ventricular septum, up into the root of the aorta, reflecting the previously freed pulmonary artery away from the surface of the aorta. Direct the knife through the aortic valve ring in the region of the commissure between anterior and left posterior valve cusps and up into the aorta.

f. Another method of opening the heart is to make a series of horizontal cuts spaced about 1 cm. apart, beginning at the apex of the heart, and continuing to the base of the papillary muscles. This method is useful in demonstrating involvement of the ventricular wall in cardiac hypertrophy or in myocardial infarction.

g. Another method of opening the heart is to make an incomplete horizontal cut on the posterior surface of the ventricles so that the apex of the heart can be flexed permitting examination of the valves from below. Continue the dissection as outlined in the "blood flow" method.

Histologic Examination

a. It is advisable to take tissue for histologic examination from the following sites:

Block I: Posterior border of left atrium toward the interatrial septum, approximately 1 cm. above the insertion of the posterior leaflet of the mitral valve.

Block II: Posterior leaflet of the mitral valve. From the slot made by removal of the left atrial block cut downward toward the apex so that the blade passes through the posterior leaflet of the mitral valve and the entire thickness of the adjacent myocardium. Extend the incision about 3 mm. below the free edge of the valve. Make a parallel cut and remove the block.

Block III: Posterior papillary muscle of the left ventricle. Make a longitudinal incision with a scalpel, starting at the apex of the posterior papillary muscle and continuing down its base. Use a parallel incision to remove the block.

Block IV: Tissue from aorta, mitral valve, and interior leaflet of mitral valve. Insert a pair of scissors beneath the anterior leaflet of the mitral valve so that one blade lies against the atrial surface of the valve and the other against the posterior (noncoronary cusp) of the aortic valve. Carry the incision upward through the middle of the posterior cusp of the aortic valve and through the lower portion of the aorta.

Make a parallel incision and remove the block.

Block V: Pulmonary artery and valve. Cut across the pulmonary artery about 1 cm. above the pulmonary valve. Make a
second incision through the center of the anterior cusp of
the pulmonary valve in the direction of the apex of the
heart, cutting through the anterior cusp, the pulmonary
arterial ring and down into the wall of the right ventricle.
Remove the block by means of a parallel incision.

Block VI: Right atrium and right ventricle. Cut through the
wall of the right atrium and septal leaflet of the tricuspid
valve about 1 cm. above the septal leaflet and 5 cm. lateral
to the septal anterior commissure. (The blade of the knife
should emerge just below the posterior cusp of the aortic
valve.) Cut downward toward the apex of the heart
through the wall of the right ventricle to a point 1 cm.
below the free edge of the valve. Make a parallel incision
approximately 2 mm. to the left, and remove the block.

Blocks VII and VIII: The auricular appendages. Cut through
the auricular appendages about 1.5 cm. from their tips.
Make a parallel incision 3 mm. medial to the first and
remove the blocks.

Block IX: Aorta. Cut the aorta transversely 1.5 cm. above the
aortic valve for a distance of 3 cm. Make a parallel incision
3 mm. above the first and remove the block.

Block X: Coronary arteries. Blocks of tissue 3 mm. in thickness are cut from both coronary arteries about 1.5 cm. from
their origin from the aortic valve.

b. When a conduction defect is suspected, histopathologic
study of the AV node, the bundle of His, and the bundle
branches is indicated . . . A block of tissue is taken and divided
into four parts . . .

c. The circumference of all four valves and the width of the
ventricles are measured. When a valve is stenosed the transverse
diameter of the ostium is measured . . .

Procedures for Certain Cardiac Conditions

a. In congenital heart disease it is preferable to leave the lungs attached to the heart since proper examination is time consuming and is best done after completion of the autopsy. The heart is dissected, unfixed according to the "blood flow" method; the entire specimen is then placed in 10 percent formalin for more detailed study after fixation.

b. When a pulmonary arterial embolus is found, its original site should be searched for in the right atrium and auricular appendage, the femoral and iliac veins, the veins of the upper and lower extremities, and the pelvic veins.

c. Air embolism in the heart can be demonstrated only at the time of autopsy, and a different method of opening the heart and great vessels is required.

(1) Venous air embolism may be associated with tubal patency test, pneumothorax, pneumoperitoneum, pneumoencephalographs, intravenous infusion, childbirth, or operations on neck and thorax. A large amount of air (100 to 150 cc.) is required to cause death; arterial air embolism to the left side of the heart tears in the lungs or pulmonary veins requires less. Air trapped in the left side of the heart may be embolic to the coronary or cerebral vessels.

(2) Expose the sternum and costal cartilages by a simple midline incision from just below the sternal notch to the symphygis pubis. This incision prevents introduction of air into the heart from severed superficial neck veins. Reflect the skin and muscles. Cut the rib cartilages laterally through the level of the second rib. Do not incise the sternoclavicular joint. Sever the diaphragm from the sternum. Lift up the sternum and break it to expose the pericardium. Ligate the aorta tightly proximal to the origin of the great vessels. Lift the pericardium from the surface of the heart and incise its anterior surface for a distance of 3 cm. Elevate the edges of the incision with forceps and inspect the contents, parietal pericardium and epicardium. In cases of fatal air embolism the right side of the heart may have a balloonlike appearance. Take cultures of the fluid in the pericardial sac to rule out post-mortem gaseous decomposition and clostridial

infections which may simulate air embolism.

(3) Fill the pericardial sac with water and submerge the heart. Make a single superficial cut across the left circumflex coronary artery and the descending branch of the left coronary artery; take care not to enter the chambers of the heart. "Milk" the left coronary arteries with the finger toward the incision; this allows air bubbles, if present, to be detected in the water. Repeat the procedure with the right coronary artery. Incise under water the right atrium, right ventricle and pulmonary artery, and exert slight pressure to release trapped pockets of air. Examine the left atrium, left ventricle, the superior vena cava, the inferior vena cava, and the pelvic veins in a similar manner.

(4) Air embolism may be differentiated from gaseous decomposition by placing air from the heart into a bottle containing alkaline two percent pyrogallol solution. Oxygen containing air stains this solution brown; gases of decomposition cause no change in color . . .

Trachea and Bronchi

a. Dissect remnants of the pericardial sac from the underlying structures to expose the trachea and main bronchi. Ordinarily the trachea is transected just below the larynx and is removed along both lungs. Open the trachea and bronchi with scissors by cutting through the posterior walls. The character of the mucosa and the presence of fluid, mucus, and foreign bodies should be noted.

b. In special cases, such as death due to drowning or aspiration of foreign bodies, or when bronchogenic carcinoma is present, the trachea and main bronchi should be opened *in situ* by cutting the anterior walls with a scalpel or scissors.

Lungs

Divide all structures at the hilum of each lung, noting the contents of the lumens of the bronchi, pulmonary arteries, and pulmonary veins as they are cut. The internal structure of the lung is best exposed by a single incision along the long axis of each lung, extending from the most lateral convexity toward the hilum. This incision should be so placed as to expose the maximal surface of each of the lobes of the lungs. Any further incisions should be made parallel to the primary incision. Open the major bronchi with scissors. Expose and examine the lymph nodes at the hilum. Examine the principal branches of the pulmonary artery and vein on the cut surface of the lung for thrombi and emboli, and open them further if necessary. Weigh each lung and select representative blocks for microscopic study. Blocks from the various lobes may be cut in distinctive shapes so as to indicate the origin of each.

Examination of the Larynx, Pharynx, Hypopharynx, Tongue, Thyroid, and Parathyroid

a. When there is extensive disease of these structures it is advantageous to remove all the neck organs as a unit. To accomplish this, the skin, together with the attached platysma muscle and portions of the pectoral muscles, is dissected from the underlying tissue and retracted as far superiorly as possible. The muscles of the neck will be exposed and enlarged cervical lymph nodes can be noted. Further dissection will reveal the submaxillary glands in the submaxillary triangles. The thyroid gland is brought into view by dissection and lateral retraction of the infrahyoid muscles. With blunt dissection each common carotid artery is dissected from the carotid sheath and retracted away from the larynx and trachea along its entire course in the neck. Avoid cutting the carotid arteries during this procedure because of their importance to proper embalming of the head. These vessels are ligated with long strings and then severed at their origins from the aortic arch on the left and the innominate artery on the right. The patency of the internal carotid arteries can be tested by injecting them with physiological solution of sodium chloride after the brain has been removed.

b. The extrinsic muscles of the tongue are cut through their attachment to the mandible and styloid process with the amputating knife. The stylopharyngeus muscle is severed from the styloid process at the same time. The soft palate and uvulva are cut from their attachments. The mobilized tongue is drawn inferiorly and the posterior wall of the pharynx and esophagus separated from the underlying tissues. The lower respiratory tract, including the trachea, bronchi, and lungs, may be left attached to the upper air passage or the trachea, while the proximal portion of the esophagus may be transected. In this way the tongue, the pharynx, the pharyngeal muscles, the larynx, the trachea, the thyroid, the parathyroids, and the proximal portion of the esophagus are removed *en bloc*. After examination of the surface of the tongue, multiple transverse sections are made.

   c. Dissection of the parathyroid glands is facilitated by removal of the new structures *en bloc* so that there will be landmarks. The parathyroids are sought from the posterior aspect. The prosector is more likely to find all parathyroid glands if he is seated and has a spotlight directed on the field. Some pathologists prefer to fix the specimen in formalin before attempting to locate the parathyroid glands, because they are firmer and a deeper yellowish brown than in the fresh state. The upper parathyroid glands are usually found embedded in the deep cervical fascia between the esophagus and the posterior aspect of the upper portions of the lateral lobes of the thyroid. The lower parathyroids are usually found in the deep cervical fascia along the inferolateral aspect of the lateral lobes of the thyroid. Occasionally the parathyroids may be embedded in the thyroid gland. The normal parathyroid glands are yellow-brown vascular structures that are distinct in color and consistency from the surrounding softer yellow fat and firmer gray lymph nodes. In cases in which the parathyroid glands are of unusual interest, all the tissue from this region should be saved for microscopic examination in the event that all the glands are not identified grossly. After the parathyroid glands are removed, the thyroid gland is dissected from the larynx and multiple sections are made through it.

   d. The upper air passage should be examined for evidence of obstruction before it is opened. Next, the hypopharynx, including the epiglottis and the pyriform sinuses, should be examined. The upper portion of the esophagus is opened posteriorly and dissected away from the posterior wall of the larynx. The larynx is then opened longitudinally along its posterior aspect to reveal the vocal cords.

Mesentery and Intestine

a. Excise the greater omentum close to its attachment to the stomach. The superior mesenteric artery and vein can be examined when the transverse colon and its mesentery are drawn superiorly. By this maneuver the root of the mesentery and its vessels will usually be exposed. In an obese subject it will be necessary to remove fat to bring the vessels to view. Open the vein and the artery. Examine the mesentery by multiple sections across the mesenteric arteries, veins, and lymph nodes. Tie the jejunum with double ligatures for a few centimeters below the ligament of Treitz. Use a sharp, long knife to separate the intestine from the mesentery as close as possible to the intestine. On reaching the ileocecal region, incise the peritoneum of the posterior abdominal wall and lift the cecum and ascending colon free from the surrounding tissues. Separate the transverse colon from its attachments to the stomach, and raise the descending colon away from the posterior abdominal wall. Displace feces from the sigmoid and rectum by stripping upward into the descending colon. Place double ligatures about the sigmoid colon 5 to 6 cm. above the sigmoidorectal junction. Cut between the double ligatures around the jejunum and colon and lift the entire intestine from the body.

b. The rectum is removed along with the bladder as . . . described under *Urinary Tract*.

c. Remove the mesentery of the small intestine by severing its attachment to the posterior abdominal wall. Open the small intestine with blunt scissors or enterotome along the mesenteric attachment, and the large intestine along one of the taenia. The appendix may be examined by multiple cross sections or by a longitudinal incision through the lumen. As the intestine is opened, note the fluidity, color, and other characteristics of its contents. Take sections of representative regions. Do not rub the fingers over the mucosa or wash it with water before the sections are placed in fixative. Record the thickness, consistency, and color of the mucosa and of the wall as a whole.

Spleen

Examine the anterior surface of the pancreas, the splenic artery, the vein on the superior surface of the body and tail of the pancreas. Lift the spleen, divide the vessels at the hilum, and remove the spleen. Weigh the organ and measure its length, breadth, and thickness. Expose the parenchyma by a single incision extending from the greatest convexity toward the hilum. Further incisions should parallel the first. Fix a representative block from the organ, including the capsule.

Gallbladder, Ducts, and Porta Hepatis

Open the first and second portions of the duodenum by an incision on the anterior surface. Locate the major and minor duodenal papillae. Exert pressure on the gallbladder and note whether bile streams from the major papilla. Divide the peritoneal covering on the lateral walls of the duodenum and expose the lower part of the common bile duct. With a scalpel open the duct, and with scissors extend the incision upward into the hepatic ducts and the cystic duct, and downward into the ampulla. Note the character of the bile in the ducts and inspect for calculi. Open the gallbladder longitudinally with scissors and collect the bile in a clean dry glass container, or the gallbladder may be dissected intact from its bed after removal of the liver, and then opened. Inspect the bile for concrements and examine the mucosa and wall of the gallbladder. Open the portal vein and the splenic veins. Examine the hepatic artery.

Esophagus, Stomach, and Duodenum

If there is no pathologic change to indicate the desirability of keeping the liver, bile ducts, and duodenum in one piece, cut across the structures in the hepatoduodenal ligament and remove the duodenum, pancreas, stomach, and esophagus *in toto*. Extend the previous incision in the anterior surface of the first part of the duodenum along the greater curvature of the stomach and up the anterior wall of the esophagus. Note the character of the stomach contents, the thickness, rugae of the mucosa, and other features of the walls. Extend the incision in the second part of the duodenum so as to open the entire length of the third part.

Pancreas

Examine the pancreas by making multiple cross sections or by a single frontal section extending from the inferior border to the superior border. On the cut surface locate the pancreatic duct; note its size and content, and the character of its wall. With small sharp-pointed scissors open the pancreatic duct. Separate the pancreas from the duodenum by dissection. Weigh it and measure the long axis, the width of the head, and the average depth. Select blocks of the head, body, and tail for microscopic study. The islands are most numerous in the tail. This block should be used for routine sections.

Liver

Remove the liver by division of the triangular ligaments and the hepatic veins as they join the inferior vena cava at the lower border of the diaphragm. Weigh the liver and measure its three principal axes. The first incision in the liver should extend on the long axis and be directed from the greater convexity toward the porta hepatis. Further incisions should be parallel to the first. Place representative blocks, including the capsule, in fixative.

Adrenal Glands

Free the adrenal glands by dissection and remove extraneous

tissue. Weigh the organs if the size is abnormal and examine the cut surface by making parallel sections. Place a part or all of each organ in 10 percent formalin.

Aorta and Vena Cava

a. Use an enterotome to open the aorta along the anterior surface. Inspect the intima, the wall, and the orifices of each of the principal branches. The orifices should be opened. If there is no pathologic change in the renal arteries or renal veins, they may be divided at a point 1 cm. from the aortic orifice. If the arch of the aorta is to be removed, the 3 major branches (innominate, left common carotid, and left subclavian arteries) must be ligated about 2 cm. above their origins and severed below the ligatures which should be left with ends at least 5 inches long for the use of embalmers.

b. Open the inferior vena cava from the bifurcation of the iliac veins to the level of the diaphragm.

Urinary Tract

Remove urine from the bladder with a syringe and needle if indicated. With a finger or blunt instrument separate the bladder from the extraperitoneal tissues of the retrosymphysial space so that the bladder and prostate are completely free from the pelvic wall. Further dissection with the fingers porteriorly will separate the rectum from the body wall. A knife or curved scissors may be used to cut the urethra distal to the prostate and the rectum not less than 2 cm. above the anorectal junction. Reflect the pelvic organs upward and outward, exposing the great iliac vessels. Free the kidneys and ureters by retracting them toward the midline from surrounding structures and remove them by a sharp dissection along with the bladder, internal genitalia, and rectum from the body in one block.

Kidneys

With a long knife divide the kidney into anterior and posterior halves by a straight, sharp, single incision along the longitudinal axis of the convexity. With scissors open the pelves and the ureters, the renal artery and vein and their major branches. Record the weight, length, breadth, and depth of each kidney after severing the ureter. Strip the capsule to expose the surface of the parenchyma. For histologic study remove a block of tissue 3 to 5 mm. thick, including cortex, medulla, and pelvic mucous membrane from each kidney . . . Measure the thickness of the cortex and the thickness of the entire renal substance.

Urinary Bladder

Open the bladder by a vertical incision on the anterior surface extending from the fundus to within a few millimeters of the internal urethral orifice. Invert and inspect the mucosa and wall. Select a block to include all layers of the wall for fixation.

Prostate

The prostate is examined by multiple coronal sections 5 to 6 mm. apart, extending from the base of the bladder to the apex of the prostate. Inspect the mucosa of the urethra. Place one complete coronal block, including the posterior lobe, in fixative.

Rectum and Sigmoid

Open the rectum with an enterotome along the posterior midline. Remove fecal material and examine the mucosa and wall. Dissect the rectum from the posterior wall of the bladder and from the prostate to display the seminal vesicles in men . . .

Seminal Vesicles

Multiple longitudinal incisions, 2 to 3 mm. apart, serve to expose the wall and the lumens of the vesicles. The thickness, the character of the wall, and the physical characteristics of the seminal fluid should be noted. Place a representative block in fixative.

Testes and Epididymides

a. Remove the testes by enlarging the inguinal canal, inverting the scrotum, and cutting the attachment of the tunica vaginalis to subcutaneous tissue of the lower part of the scrotum. If there are related pathologic changes in the genital tract, the testes should be mobilized before the pelvic organs are removed, so that the entire length of the vasa and the attachment to both the epididymides and the seminal vesicles are preserved.

b. Open the tunica vaginalis and note the amount and physical characteristics of the fluid it contains. Incise testes and epididymes. If abnormality exists, record the weight and measurements. Observe the thickness of the tunica, the tissues of the epididymis, and the consistency of the testis. With forceps determine the ease with which the tubules "string" from the cut surface of the testis. Place a block from the opposite half in fixative.

Vas Deferens

Examine the vas deferens by multiple cross sections without completely dividing the structure. Note the size and richness of the pampiniform plexus and inspect for thrombi.

Removal and Examination of the Brain

a. When bacteriologic or viral studies of brain tissue are indicated by clinical history or gross appearances, the brain should be removed prior to embalming . . .

b. After examination of the scalp, an intermastoidal incision extending over the vertex of the skull is made with the blade of the scalpel turned outward to prevent cutting the hair. If the subject is bald, the incision should be placed as far posteriorly as possible and may sometimes be hidden by making the incision backward from points about 2 inches above the ear to encircle the scalp posteriorly within the hairline. It is advisable to start the incision behind the right ear and end it behind the left, so that if disfigurement occurs, it will be on the left side of the head. Embalmers regard the right side of the face as the "show" side. Reflect the scalp anteriorly to a line 1.5 cm. above the supra-orbital ridge and posteriorly below the occiput. With a sharp instrument mark out the anterior saw cut from behind the ears over the frontal bone and, whenever possible, posterior to the hairline. The posterior cut should extend backward from the lower end of the anterior cut over the occipital bone to the midline at the level of the superior nuchal line, where it should meet with the posterior cut from the other side. The angle formed by the anterior and posterior skull incisions should be from 100° to 120° and should be so placed that neither limb, if extended, will intersect the external ear. This is of practical importance in protecting the ear from the saw. Use a scalpel to cut the temporal muscle and fascia along the plotted lines, and with a blunt instrument separate the tissues from the bone along the incision. Cut the entire thickness of the skull with a fine tooth saw or Stryker® saw but do not allow the saw to slip into the brain. If there is a question of possible skull fracture, do not use hammer and chisel in removing the calvaria, as these implements may create fracture lines that will complicate medicolegal cases. Remove the calvaria, separating it from the underlying dura by blunt dissection between bone and dura. Open the superior longitudinal sinus. Cut the dura with scissors along the edges of the bone and reflect it toward the midline. Use scissors to cut the falx cerebri anteriorly in the great cerebral fissure and pull the dura posteriorly, cutting the cerebral veins as necessary and the great cerebral vein of Galen in the pineal fossa. With the left hand lift the frontal lobes and olfactory nerves from the floor of the anterior fossa and use scissors to cut the optic nerves that can be reached. Place the left hand beneath the parietal lobes to support the weight of the brain and cut the tentorium cerebelli on each side beneath and close to its peripheral attachments. The posterior cranial fossa is exposed and the remaining cranial nerves and the vertebral arteries can be severed. Support the brain carefully with slight traction on the cerebral peduncles and transect the cervical cord as far inferiorly as possible. Remove the brain by lifting it with the fingers of both hands to prevent damage to the soft organ.

c. After removal, fix the brain and spinal cord in 10 percent formalin. Before the brain is placed in fixative, the corpus callosum may be incised sagittally on each side of the midline to permit access of fluid to the ventricles. Suspend the brain in a gallon jar of fixative by a string passing under the basilar artery and attached to the edges of the container. The brain should be allowed to harden in fixative for at least one week, preferably two weeks, before sectioning. The fixing fluid should be changed during the first 24 hours and at the end of one week. If immediate diagnosis is necessary, the brain may be cut in the fresh state. This procedure is expedited if the freshly sectioned surface is pressed firmly against a piece of glass before the next cut is made, and the knife blade is flooded with 95 percent alcohol. If desired, the intact fixed brain may be forwarded to the Armed Forces Institute of Pathology.

d. When the brain has hardened in fixative it should be cut in coronal sections not more than 1 cm. in thickness. Place the brain on a dissecting board with the ventral surface upward so that the landmarks of the base can be used in orienting the coronal cuts symmetrically. Remove the brain stem and cerebellum with a thin knife, cutting across the cerebral peduncles in a plane perpendicular to the axis of the brain stem and aqueduct. Begin the parallel coronal sections of the cerebral hemispheres at the frontal poles. The brain stem and cerebellum together are cut by parallel sections 0.5 cm. apart in a plane perpendicular to the axis of the brain stem.

Examination of the Base of the Skull

a. Fractures of the Base. For demonstration of fractures the dura should be stripped from the bone. This is best done by winding it onto a hemostat attached to the cut edge of the dura. Some pathologists prefer to use "gas pliers". In either case the dura should be stripped immediately after the brain is removed and before chisel and hammer are used, since they may cause fractures.

b. Pituitary Gland. The posterior clinoid processes are broken with a chisel directed toward the occiput. The diaphragm of the sella is incised around its periphery and the pituitary gland is removed by sharp dissection. The entire gland is fixed in 10 percent formalin. Later it may be sectioned either horizontally, which exposes the topographic features of the anterior lobe, or saggitally, which better demonstrates the stalk and intermediate lobe.

c. Dural Sinuses, Carotid Arteries, and Gasserian Ganglia. The dural sinuses, notably the cavernous, superior and inferior petrosal, saggital and sigmoidal, are opened with curved scissors. The carotid arteries may be traced through the walls of the cavernous sinus and in their canals by use of heavy scissors and a narrow chisel. If there is history of cerebral dysfunction, the patency of the carotids should be tested by slowly injecting saline solution into the common carotids and observing its flow out of the intracranial ends of the internal carotids. Formalin should not be used, because it might harden the features before the embalmer can "set" them. Water is inadvisable, because it may lake blood in the tissue and produce foci of discoloration. Remove the gasserian ganglia from the subdural pockets lateral to the cavernous sinus and place in 10 percent formalin.

d. Temporal Bone and Middle Ear.

    (1) To remove the temporal bone in one piece, make four primary cuts in the bone with a motor driven circular saw, or a Stryker cast cutter with a one to two inch blade. If neither of these instruments is available, a thin-bladed osteotome or a chisel and light hammer can be used. The dura should be left attached and care should be taken to remove the temporal bone in such a manner that the external contour or the head is maintained.

    (2) ... The *first* incision is placed as close as possible to the inner surface of the squamous portion of the temporal bone and directed slightly lateralward so as to include the ear drum. The *second* incision is roughly

parallel to the first and medial to the inner lip of the internal auditory meatus. The *third* incision is made about 2.5 cm. anterior to the petrous ridge. It is most important that the lateral end of this third incision be deep and connect with the first. The *fourth* incision is an undercut at the line of the inferior petrosal sinus. After the initial incisions have been made the specimen is loosened further by using a short thin-bladed osteotome in the corners and on the styloid process. When the specimen can be lifted, the attached soft tissues are severed with strong, curved scissors. When disease of the eustachian tube is suspected, the third and fourth incisions can be extended to include the sella turcica and the upper part of the nasopharynx in the block with the temporal bone. The base of the skull is weakened by removal of these bones; therefore, the fragile bridge of the temporal bones remaining laterally must be handled gently and the entire base of the skull filled with plaster of Paris to fix the anterior and posterior halves together before the calvaria is replaced.

(3) The temporal bone should be placed immediately in 500 cc. of 10 percent formalin and the fluid changed daily for 3 days before shipment.

e. *Eyes.*

(1) Either the entire eye or the posterior half of the globe may be obtained from within the cranial cavity *(special permission required).* After removing the brain and pituitary, unroof the orbit and expose the optic nerve and eyeball. Make traction on the extraocular muscles during the dissection to avoid crushing the nerve and eyeball. If the entire globe is removed, caution must be observed to avoid damage to the lids. Dissect the bulbar conjunctiva away from the globe, keeping the knife close to the corneoscleral limbus. The embalmer must be advised to suture the lids and restore the orbit.

(2) Fix the eye and attached optic nerve in 300 to 500 cc. neutral 10 percent formalin. It is not necessary to open the globe since aqueous formalin will penetrate the

sclera and effect good fixation of the retina. After fixation, the eye should be opened with a double-edged razor blade in a horizontal plane so that the macula may be sectioned in line with the optic nerve and pupil.

f. *Paranasal Sinuses.*

(1) The bony plates separating the cranial cavity from the frontal, ethmoidal, and sphenoidal sinuses may be removed by means of a chisel, and the mucosa and cavities of these structures examined. The posterior nasopharnyx and even the maxillary sinuses can be approached by a coronal incision just anterior to the sella turcica. This is followed by posterior reflection of the clivus after it has been freed by a horizontal incision above the foramen magnum and lateral incisions through the apices of the petrous processes of the temporal bones. This procedure should be used with care, for it may cause collapse of the head and face, particularly if the temporal bones have been removed.

(2) After all required structures have been removed from the cranium, ligation of the carotid and vertebral arteries will prevent seepage of embalming fluid. Since the stumps of the terminal portions of the internal carotid arteries are frequently too short for satisfactory ligation, the dura covering the trigeminal ganglion lateral to the sella turcica is avulsed, thus uncovering the sigmoid portion of the internal carotid arteries. The skin flaps of the scalp should be restored to their natural positions to avoid creasing of the forehead.

Cisternal Puncture

a. The head is placed in a true lateral position and flexed maximally. Stabilize this position. The needle must be inserted just above the spine of the second vertebra, held at that point by the thumb, and then directed upward in the midline, using the top of the auricle (external ear) as a guide. The needle will usually touch the occiput, but by repeatedly withdrawing it slightly and depressing the point a little at a time it will enter the cisterna magna at such an angle that there is a distance of 2 to 3 cm. between the site of entry and the medulla. The distance from the skin to the cisterna varies, but in adults it is usually 4 to 5 cm. and *seldom* over 6 cm.

b. In some cases it may be more convenient to remove fluid by spinal puncture in the conventional manner.

Removal and Examination of the Spinal Cord

a. Approach. The spinal cord can be removed from the posterior or anterior approach. The posterior approach allows complete exposure of the spinal cord *in situ,* the spinal canal, the intervertebral foramina, and the roots and ganglia of the spinal nerves. The anterior route is less laborious, does not require an additional skin incision, and gives easier and more satisfactory exposure of the lumbar cord and cauda equina but usually does not permit one to obtain the dura mater or nerve roots above the tenth thoracic vertebra.

b. Posterior Removal. The body is placed prone on the table, with a block beneath the thorax to arch the thoracic spine. The head is placed over the edge of the table with the face protected by a sponge or towel from deforming pressure. A skin incision is made in the midline from the base of the skull to the sacrum; the paraspinal muscles are retracted laterally and the spinous processes and laminae scraped clean of muscle and fascia. The laminae, close to the spinous processes are cut with single or double bladed saw or with a specially devised chisel. If they are not entirely cut through, use a hammer and chisel to complete the separation. The spinous processes and adjacent laminae are removed en masse. A laminectomy should not be done on the first cervical vertebra as it will destroy the rigidity of the connection between the head and the trunk. The spinal cord encased in its dura mater is removed by cutting the spinal nerves lateral to the posterior root ganglia and freeing the epidural tissue by sharp dissection. The cord may be damaged if it is pulled or bent to free it from the spinal canal. A better method is to make traction in the line of the longitudinal axis of the cord by grasping the dura with forceps and exerting gentle force inferiorly. The dura is opened with scissors along the posterior or anterior midline and the cord is fixed by suspending it in a tall jar of 10 percent formalin, or by pinning the opened dura to a strip of wood in a long narrow covered dish (catheter tray) containing 10 percent formalin. Examination of the cord is made by means of multiple cross sections. Blocks for microscopic study are taken at appropriate levels.

 c. Anterior Removal. (Method of Kernohan) Following removal of the brain the upper cervical nerve roots are cut intradurally with a long narrow bladed knife as far inferiorly as possible. After the viscera have been removed from the thorax and abdomen, the bodies of the vertebrae are freed from the attachments of the psoas muscle and ligaments. The vertebral column is cut longitudinally with a round-end saw or with the large blade of an electric saw. The incision should be placed about 1 cm. to the right of the subject's midline and directed to the left at an angle of about 30° to enter the left side of the spinal canal as indicated in figure 15. The incision should start at the promontory of the sacrum and continue upward through the tenth thoracic vertebra or higher. The pedicles on the right are cut beneath the vertebral bodies with heavy bone cutting forceps or a chisel. The intervertebral discs at the upper and lower ends of the segment are removed by cutting with a knife. The broad chisel is driven into the saw cut to free the wedge-shaped segment of vertebral column. The anterior surface of the dura mater, the nerve roots, the dorsal root ganglia of the lumbar cord and the cauda equina are exposed. The spinal nerves are cut as far laterally as possible and the dura mater is cut completely around at its upper level of exposure. If the brain is not to be removed, the cord is cut as high as possible in the thorax of neck by inserting a narrow knife through an intervertebral disc. The cord may then be removed by exerting gentle traction on the dura. Restoration of the vertebral column seldom is necessary because sufficient rigidity is maintained by the remaining parts.

Examination of Specific Peripheral Nerves and Neuromuscular Apparatus

When indicated, the peripheral nerves and the muscles they supply should be removed through longitudinal incisions in the skin (*special permission required*). Blocks of nerve tissue should be removed above and below the lesions and fixed in 10 percent formalin. Each block should be tagged individually or placed in a separate bottle of fixative with an identifying label.

Bones, Cartilages, Joints, and Bone Marrow

Whenever skeletal or joint disease is known or suspected roentgenograms should be obtained or consulted to aid in the selection of material. In many cases it is advisable to obtain the consent of the next-of-kin and to consult with the mortician before removing bones or joints. The mortician may wish to do part of the embalming before or during the autopsy. Bones or cartilage for grafting should be taken only from certain types of cadavers and the details and technique of selection should be discussed with the clinician who has requested the material.

Ribs

The study of nutritional deficiencies, metabolic derangements and other effects on osseous and cartilaginous growth may require the removal of several costochondral junctions. These should be split or sawed longitudinally before fixation.

Calvaria

In certain anemias infections and other diseases, it is desirable to sample the calvaria. This can be done by removing bone from between two closely placed parallel saw cuts.

Digits

The small bones and joints of the hands and feet can be

removed through palmar or plantar longitudinal incisions. The skeletal contours can be restored if necessary by inserting wooden substitutes for the resected bones. Special permission is necessary.

Extremities

a. The humerus may be reached through the usual **Y**-shaped body incision by cutting across the muscles of the anterior part of the axilla. The brachial vessels need not be severed. No additional skin incision is necessary unless the whole humerus is to be removed. If the capsule is opened the head of the humerus can be delivered by anterior dislocation. The muscle attachments can be progressively dissected away to the desired level. A small wooden rod, cut to the desired length, can be driven into the marrow cavity of the distal portion of the humerus and fixed to the acromion by means of a previously inserted nail (the head of a nail is sawed off and its blunt end driven into one end of the wooden rod). The proximal end of the rod is then wired to the glenoid fossa.

b. The femur can be delivered through an anteromedial incision in Scarpa's triangle cutting through the inguinal ligament and extending the skin incision for a few inches. After the anterior group of muscles is severed, the muscle attachments of the greater trochanter are cut away, the capsule and ligmentum teres are incised and the head of the femur is dislocated anteriorly. Muscle attachments to the shaft are then removed progressively, while traction is exerted on the head. The femur can be transected at the desired level and replaced with a wooden rod driven into the distal marrow cavity. The proximal end of the rod in which a nail has been fixed is pushed into the roof of the scetabulum. Unless the rod is somewhat longer than the portion of femur removed, it will be easily dislodged when the body is moved. A segment of cortex and bone marrow can be removed from the shaft . . .

Knee Joint

The knee joint can be exposed by an anterior curved incision immediately below the patella. Flex the knee and carry the incision through the quadriceps tendon to expose the joint. To dislocate the joint, cut the capsule and cruciate ligaments and free the muscle attachments. Tissue from the articular surfaces, joint capsule, bursae, and tendon may be obtained. If the knee joint is to be removed as a unit, a longitudinal anteromedial incision is employed. The distal portion of the incision should be well above the hemline of the dress to be worn. The cooperation of the mortician is essential for this procedure, since loss of contour is inevitable. Prosthesis may be accomplished by driving a wooden rod into the cut end of the shaft of the femur and proximal tibia.

Sternoclavicular Joints

The sternoclavicular joints are readily removed and offer an opportunity for the simultaneous examination of bone and joint. Prosthesis is generally unnecessary except occasionally to restore contour in women.

Vertebrae

The vertebrae can usually be satisfactorily examined either by removing the anterior halves of the bodies by means of a coronal saw cut or by inspecting the blocks obtained in removing the spinal cord by the anterior route. If the vertebral column must be removed, the best approach is anteriorly from within the body cavity. Divide the soft tissues of the posterior abdominal wall where they attach to the vertebrae and transect the ribs near the transverse processes. Cut the intervertebral discs at the lowest and highest points of the selected specimen and dissect the bony mass from the body. The rigidity of the vertebral column should be restored by use of a stick of wood. Metal should be avoided in restoration, especially if the body is to be cremated.

Bone Marrow

Bone marrow may be obtained by the following methods:

a. Saw through the anterior one-third of a vertebra to expose the bone marrow. Dig out a block of bone marrow with a cartilage knife and place in 90 cc. of Zenker's fluid to which 10 cc. of glacial acetic acid has been added, for 24 hours. Wash in running tap water for 24 hours. Usually sufficient decalcification of the cancellous bone will have taken place to permit embedding and sectioning.

b. Scoop bone marrow from the femur from the incision . . .

c. Resect a segment of rib and squeeze out bone marrow by compressing the rib with a pair of pliers. Make smears on cover slips and slides and stain by Wright's method or with Giemsa stain after fixation for 2 minutes in absolute methyl alcohol. Dilute the bone marrow with an equal amount of serum to obtain thin spreads.

Examination of the Tissues of the Arm and Hand

A cardinal principle in all autopsies is that the skin of the face, the neck, the arms, and the hands must not be incised without *specific permission*. If the structures within the arm or hand must be examined, it is sometimes convenient to make a complete circular incision through the skin of the upper arm, and invert and roll the skin downward until the region to be examined is reached.

Examination of Tissues of the Face

Examination of the underlying tissues of the face should *not* be performed without *special permission* and important indication. None but the most expert should attempt this examination. The procedure is based upon the following steps; preparation of a death mask, thorough embalming and hardening of the skin and subcutaneous tissues, dissection of these tissues from the underlying bone, and final restoration by placing the embalmed skin in the death mask and recasting the facial features with plaster of Paris behind the skin.

STANDARDS FOR THE MEDICAL-LEGAL
INVESTIGATION OF DEATH*

Leslie I. Lukash, M.D.

(Chief Medical Examiner, Nassau County, New York)

On the stage of life the physician has many roles and many opportunities. He or she may be a counselor, therapist, surgeon, psychiatrist, gynecologist, internist, orthopedist or pediatrician; the list extends to the limits of peoples' needs and infirmities. Yet, the physician also has a role in death.

As a former president of the National Association of Medical Examiners and as a person who has spent his professional life in the practice of pathology and forensic pathology, I have found that the medical examiner who is charged with the responsibility of investigating violent, sudden and suspicious death, has as much a responsibility in caring for the dead as the physician who cares for the living. The examiner is a vital part of our modern medico-legal investigative system, concerned with the health and safety of people as well as the preservation of the judicial system.

The medical examiner's investigation is comprised of an examination of the scene of death and a thorough postmortem examination, including a complete autopsy and the use of all laboratory aids available in establishing and certifying the cause and manner of death. The complexity and sophistication of these procedures vary in different situations, as they do in any diagnostic attempt by a physician to establish a competent cause of a patient's complaint.

As the official responsible for the results and interpretations of all examinations in the institution, the fulfillment of the obligation entailed in this affinity is a burdensome sense of responsibility. This function directly affects each of the decedents and survivors, along with the entire community, and, as such, is a professional act requiring a physician skilled not only in medical and laboratory practices, but also with experience and knowledge in the medico-legal investigation of

---

*(From Leslie I. Lukash, Standards for the Medical-Legal Investigation of Death, *Tulane Medicine*, 6 and 7, Nos. 2 and 3:4-5, 1974. Courtesy of publisher.)

death.

The medical examiner is duly charged with the solicitude for the bereaved and with painstaking concern for the public good. The medical examiner must use all the training and experience of pathology, as well as that of toxicology, serology, anthropology and other related disciplines, to assist him in establishing a diagnosis of death.

Most deaths that fall under the jurisdiction of the medical examiner are reported by physicians, hospital personnel, law enforcement agencies and private citizens. The types of death are those that fall in the category of unnatural or suspicious death, and are ones which doctors are unable to certify as naturally caused.

As soon as the death is reported, the medical examiner, or his designee, assumes charge of the investigation. He or she examines the body and investigates the scene where the body is found.

When there is a question of criminality, the body and scene should be examined by a forensic pathologist. Whenever a question of criminality occurs, extensive procedures become not a matter of course, but rather a matter of concern to the whole community, and as such are performed within the statutes that govern the medical examiner.

Within these procedures are:

1. Determining the cause, manner and estimated time of death.
2. Recovering, identifying and preserving evidentiary material.
3. Providing interpretation and correlation of facts related to death.
4. Preserving a factual, subjective medical report for law enforcement, prosecution and defense agencies.
5. Separating natural deaths from unnatural deaths for protection of the innocent in suspicious cases.

The preliminary procedures require:

1. Examination of the body before removal of clothing to note the condition of the clothing and to correlate defects and tears with obvious injuries and to record artifacts.

2. Protection of clothing, body and hands against possible contamination prior to subsequent specific examination.
3. Recording of the general state of the body and clothing.
4. Observation of the extent of rigor mortis and lividity.
5. Recording of the temperature of the body and environment and any other data pertinent to subsequent determination of the time of death.
6. Notation of the date, time and place of the autopsy procedure, the name of the examiner.
7. Notation of observers present.
8. Photographs used to identify the body and for reference in identifying specific injuries; also, to demonstrate and to correlate external injuries with internal injuries.
9. Use of X-ray, which is important in locating bullets or other radiopaque objects for identification of the victim and for documentation of old fractures or anatomical deformities such as metallic foreign plates, nails, screws.
10. Labeling all evidentiary items, such as bullets, pellets, etc. for proper identification.
11. Preserving all tissue, fluids, and hair samples for further histological, bacteriological, histochemical, chemical and toxicological examination.

It is important to preserve all records so that copies are available to the prosecuting attorney in potential criminal investigation and to other interested parties, such as insurance companies. If litigation is pending, the defense attorney, in both civil and criminal cases, is afforded similar opportunities.

The procedures I have outlined, which are followed conscientiously by medical examiners, partially describe the integral part of our profession. The medical examiner's concern and responsibility to the deceased is no less than the practitioner's concern for the care of the living. Both serve mankind in several manners for the improvement of society, our way of life, and life itself.

The bereaved relatives, the public health and safety, the courts of our land and, perhaps even the lives and liberty of accused people, all rely upon the integrity of our function.

The family of the dead merits our assiduous concern in determining the most accurate cause and manner of death. The courts must be served with the same objective interest. The medical examiner's adherence to true findings must be based upon all the scientific means available and must be unremitting.

Innocence or guilt, malpractice or negligence, accident or purposeful: the determination of these queries are all within the realm of our responsibility.

The forensic scientist and pathologist approaches his work with the full realization that the autopsy must be supplemented by careful investigation, including a study of the background of the deceased, the circumstances under which death took place, and examination of the place of death.

After the autopsy, chemical tests, histological, serological, bacteriological, hematological, radiological, retrospective and psychiatric evaluations are important, almost as important as the autopsy itself. It is evident that at times the autopsy is only a means to an end.

All of the examinations and tests utilized by the medical examiner in the care of the dead are utilized in a similar way in the care of the living. In fact, the medical examiner's responsibility for the care of the dead and the physician's responsibility for the care of the living are similar in a way, since both are diagnosticians. The medical examiner diagnoses the death as to cause and manner and the physician diagnoses the cause of illness for possible further treatment.

The routine examination, with all the necessary ancillary diagnostic procedures, must be performed on the dead just as the routine examination and its many diagnostic tests and consultations are performed on the living to establish a diagnosis.

None of us is clairvoyant to the extent that we can arrive at a cause of death without a comprehensive approach based upon the scientific means at our disposal.

Standards for the care of the dead must be established where they do not exist. The means for this accomplishment would be to set such standards for accreditation of the medical examiner's office. These would be similar to the system of accreditation by the joint commission of accreditation of facilities in the care of the living.

Today we well know that there is no uniformity; and where there is no uniformity or living up to standards such as we espouse, there can be no quality of professionalism.

There is a task before us, as I see it ... to establish, by accreditation, uniformity of standards for the care of the dead on a national scale. Accreditation is the only possible answer to insure national standards in the medico-legal investigation of death.

PHOTOGRAPHIC AND X-RAY MATERIALS

$\mathbf{P}$RESUMABLY photographs were taken at the J.F. Kennedy autopsy. X-ray films were exposed. The evidence seems clear that the pathologists saw some of the x-rays on the night of the autopsy. It is not clear that they ever saw all the photographs.

Several inventories of photo materials and x-rays were made. They do not agree. This Appendix lists the inventories made. The validity of any of them is problematical. The chain of custody of each individual item is questionable. The probative value of these materials is probably of low order: Too much in the way of surreptitious manipulations casts a deep shadow of doubt on the authenticity of the material.

FBI ORIGINAL INVENTORY

The FBI report (Commission Document No. 7) gives an inventory of x-rays and photographs made at the autopsy.

11 x-rays
22 4″ x 5″ color photographs
18 4″ x 5″ black and white photographs
1 roll of 120 film containing five exposures

The x-rays were said to have been developed at the hospital; the photographs were turned over undeveloped to the Secret Service.

It seems apparent that the pathologists were in a position to validate the x-rays. They could not validate the photographs because they never saw them. The peculiar handling of this autopsy material is impossible to explain in any rational way.

The end result of the unprofessional, unconventional manner of handling illustrations of the autopsy is to make it forever impossible to reconstruct with reliability the truth of the postmortem examinations.

TECHNICAL PROBLEMS

Some filing problems as well as the quality of the films obviously have arisen with the x-ray films. A few examples will suffice to illustrate the matter.

- X-ray film number 2, 8 x 10 inches, in 1966 was said to be right side of skull (Humes et al., 1966, p. 2). In 1968, a special panel called it a left side of skull view (Carnes et al., 1968, p. 5).
- Photographs that should portray the inside of the skull cavity to illustrate the damage done by the shooting were of a quality that has been described as lacking clarity and detail (Carnes et al., 1968, p. 5).
- Heat damage has been found on x-ray number 1; pencil marks are reported on x-ray number 2.
- No trace can be found of x-rays of the head or identification photographs made before the anatomical dissection was begun. Were they taken? If so, were they lost or destroyed?
- Several inventories of the autopsy materials conflict with one another. Of primary concern has been the absence of the brain, microscope slides of the skin and brain, as well as photographs of the interior of the three body cavities — head, thorax, abdomen.
- Apparently Admiral Burkley filed an inventory of autopsy materials on 26 April 1965. It seems to be "classified" and is not available for scholarly study. That fact arouses additional suspicions of "doctored" evidence files.

INVENTORY OF AUTOPSY FILMS

Commission Report 26 November 1963		New York Times 29 October 1966	
Negative Type	Number	Negative Type	Number
x-ray	1	x-ray	1
	2	10 x 12 inches	2
	3		3
	4		4
	5		5
	6		6
	7	x-ray	7
	8	14 x 17 inches	8
	9		9
	10		10
	11		11
			12*
			13*
			14*
Black and white 4 x 5 inches	1	Black and white negatives	1
	2		2
	3		3
	4		4
	5		5
	6		6
	7		7
	8		8
	9		9
	10		10
	11		11
	12		12
	13		13
	14		14
	15		15
	16		16
	17		17
	18		18

*Missing from 26 November 1963 inventory.

26 November 1963		*29 October 1966*	
Negative Type	*Number*	*Negative Type*	*Number*
		Black and white	19
		4 x 5 inches†	20
			21
			22
			23
			24
			25
Color	1	Color	1
4 x 5 inches	2	transparency	2
	3	4 x 5 inches	3
	4		4
	5		5
	6		6
	7		7
	8		8
	9		9
	10		10
	11		11
	12		12
	13		13
	14		14
	15		15
	16		16
	17		17
	18		18
	19		19
	20		20
	21		21
	22		22
	‡		23
			24
			25
			26
			27

†During examination of the brain on 6 December 1963 seven black and white negatives were exposed (Commission Exhibit No. 391, vol. XVI, p. 988).

‡During examination of the brain on 6 December 1963 six color 4 x 5 inch negatives were exposed (Commission Exhibit No. 391, vol. XVI, p. 988). There were only five on 29 October 1966.

Negative Type	Number	Negative Type	Number
		Film 4 x 5 inches§	1 2 3 4 5
		Color film§	1 roll
		Color film‖	1 piece
120 film§	1 2 3 4 5		
Total "A complete listing" according to FBI (Commission Document No. 7, p. 285).	56	Total Negatives and transparencies Roll of film (*New York Times*, 6 January 1968, pp. 1, 15).	72

§Exposed, no image.
‖Unexposed.

In the explicit language of their agreement with the government, the Kennedy's turned over ". . . certain x-rays and photographs connected with the autopsy. . ." These were not *all* the films (*New York Times*, 6 January 1967, p. 15).

INVENTORY

1 November 1966

Negative Type	Number	ID Number	Description	Comments
x-ray 8 x 10 inches	1	21296	SKULL: front-back view	". . .slight heat damaged. . ."
	2	21296	SKULL: side, right view	". . .two angle lines over-drawn on the film. . ."
	3	21296	SKULL: side view	
	4	None	BONE fragment	Numbers 1-6: 10 x 12 inches on
	5	None	BONE fragment	29 October 1966
	6	None	BONE fragment	
x-ray 14 x 17 inches	7	21296	ABDOMEN: front-back view	
	8	21296	SHOULDER, right; CHEST, right	front-back view
	9	21296	CHEST: front-back view	
	10	21296	SHOULDER, left; CHEST, left	front-back view
	11	21296	CHEST, lower; ABDOMEN	front-back view
	12	21296	THIGHS, both; KNEE JOINTS, both	front-back view
	13	21296	PELVIS: front-back view	". . .a small round density of myelogram media pro-jected over the sacral canal. . ."
	14	21296	PELVIS, lower; HIPS and THIGHS, upper, front-back view	
Black and white negatives 4 x 5 inches	1		HEAD, left; SHOULDERS	
	2		Similar	
	3		Similar	
	4		Similar	
	5		HEAD, right; SHOULDER, right	
	6		Similar	
	7		HEAD, above	
	8		Similar	
	9		Similar	
	10		Similar	
	11		SHOULDER wound, back view	
	12		Similar	
	13		HEAD, front; TORSO, upper	Shows tracheotomy wound.

Negative Type	Number	ID Number	Description	Comments
	14		Similar	". . .somewhat closer view. . ."
	15		SKULL, wound, right, rear	occipital area
	16		Similar	
	17		Similar	shows wound ". . .following reflection of scalp. . ."
	18		Similar	
	19	JTB	BRAIN, below	
	20	JTB	BRAIN, above	
	21	JTB	BRAIN, below	
	22	JTB	BRAIN	". . .direct basilar view. . ."
	23	JTB	BRAIN, above	Shows ". . .extensive damage to right cerebral hemisphere. . ."
	24	JTB	Similar	
	25	JTB	Similar	
Color trans- parencies 4 x 5 inches	26		HEAD, right side	
	27		Similar	
	28		Similar	
	29		HEAD, left side	
	30		Similar	
	31		Similar	
	32		HEAD, above	
	33		Similar	
	34		Similar	
	35		Similar	
	36		Similar	
	37		Similar	
	38		SHOULDER, wound, right, upper back	
	39		SHOULDER, wound, right, upper back	
	40		HEAD and TORSO, upper front	Shows tracheotomy wound
	41		Similar	
	42		HEAD, wound, right occipital area	
	43		Similar	
	44		HEAD, wound, back	". . .with scalp reflected. . ."
	45		Similar	
	46		BRAIN, below	
	47		Similar	
	48		Similar	
	49		Color negative; no transparency	Made from 47, which has better

Negative Type	Number	ID Number	Description	Comments
			Has brush hair	color intensity
	50		BRAIN, above	
	51		Similar	
	52		Similar	Now seven brain pictures
Black and	1		Unexposed	Kennedys claim exposed
white	2		Unexposed	Developed
negatives	3		Unexposed	Developed
4 x 5	4		Unexposed	Developed
inches	5		Unexposed	Developed
Ekta-chrome® Film 4 x 5 inches			Unexposed	Undeveloped
Ekta-chrome Trans-parency 4 x 5 inches	1		Unexposed	Developed
120 Color Film	roll		No recognizable image	Processed. Secret Service seized and exposed it to light.
Total	72 Negatives and transparencies 2 Rolls of film			

(Humes et al., 1966)

INVENTORY

26-27 February 1968

Negative Type	Number	ID Number	Description	Comments
x-ray	1	21296	SKULL: front-back view	possible heat damage in two small areas.

Negative Type	Number	ID Number	Description	Comments
2		21296	SKULL: left side	Right side in November 1966. Shows rear hole 4 inches high. Converging pencil lines drawn on film.
3		21296	SKULL: left side	Slightly different projection.
4		21296	SKULL fragments	
5		21296	SKULL fragments	
6		21296	SKULL fragments	
7		21296	CHEST and STOMACH: front-back view	
8		21296	CHEST, right; SHOULDER and ARM, upper, front-back view	Lower neck can be seen
9		21296	CHEST: front-back view	Lower neck can be seen
10		21296	CHEST, left; SHOULDER and ARM, upper, front-back view	Lower neck can be seen
11		21296	CHEST and STOMACH: front-back view	
12		21296	THIGHS, lower; KNEES: front-back	
13		21296	PELVIS: front-back view	". . .a small, round opaque structure. . .1 mm in diameter. . .to the right of the midline at. . .the first sacral segment of the spine."
14			LEGS, upper, front-back view	
18	1 JB		HEAD and NECK, left side	
17	2 JB		HEAD and NECK, left side	
6	3 JB		HEAD and NECK, left side	
15	4 JB		HEAD and NECK, left side	
12	5 JB		HEAD, right, above; part of FACE, NECK, SHOULDER, and CHEST, upper	
11	6 JB		HEAD, right, above; part of FACE, NECK, SHOULDER, and CHEST, upper	
8	7 JB		HEAD, above	
13	8 JB		HEAD, above	
5	9 JB		HEAD, above	
16	10 JB		HEAD, above	
9	11 JB		BACK and NECK	
10	12 JB		BACK and NECK	
4	13 JB		HEAD, right, above; part of	

Negative Type	Number	ID Number	Description	Comments
	3	14 JB	FACE, NECK, SHOULDER, and CHEST, upper HEAD, right, above; part of FACE, NECK, SHOULDER, and CHEST, upper	
	14	15 JB	HEAD, back	
	7	16 JB	HEAD, back	
	2	17 JB	CRANIAL CAVITY, above, above, brain removed	*Lack of contrast and clarity of detail*
	1	18 JB	CRANIAL CAVITY, above, front, brain removed	*Lack of contrast and clarity of detail*
Black and white negatives		19 JTB	BRAIN	*Gray brown rectangular structure, 13 x 20 mm present. Not noted in previous inventories.*
		20 JTB	BRAIN	
		21 JTB	BRAIN	
		22 JTB	BRAIN	
		23 JTB	BRAIN	
		24 JTB	BRAIN	
		25 JTB	BRAIN	
	26		HEAD, right, above; part of FACE, NECK, SHOULDER, and CHEST, upper	
	27		HEAD, right, above; part of FACE, NECK, SHOULDER, and CHEST, upper	
	28		HEAD, right, above; part of FACE, NECK, SHOULDER, and CHEST, upper	
	29		HEAD and NECK, left side	
	30		HEAD and NECK, left side	
	31		HEAD and NECK, left side	
	32		HEAD, above	
	33		HEAD, above	
	34		HEAD, above	
	35		HEAD, above	
	36		HEAD, above	
	37		HEAD, above	
	38		BACK and NECK	
	39		BACK and NECK	
	40		HEAD, right, above; part of FACE, NECK, SHOULDER, and CHEST, upper	
	41		HEAD, right, above; part of FACE, NECK, SHOULDER, and CHEST, upper	
	42		HEAD, back	

Negative Type	Number	ID Number	Description	Comments
	43		HEAD, back	
	44		CRANIAL CAVITY, above, front brain removed	*Lack of contrast and clarity of detail*
	45		CRANIAL CAVITY, above, front brain removed	*Lack of contrast and clarity of detail*
	46		BRAIN, below	*Gray brown rectangular structure,*
	47		BRAIN, below	*13 x 20 mm present. Not noted*
	48		BRAIN, below	*in previous inventories.*
	49		BRAIN, below	
	50		BRAIN, above	
	51		BRAIN, above	
	52		BRAIN, above	

Total 66 Negatives

(Carnes et al., 1968)

BIBLIOGRAPHY

Adelson, L. 1961. A microscopic study of dermal gunshot wounds. *Am J Clin Pathol* 35:393-402.

Alvarez, L. W. 1976. A physicist examines the Kennedy assassination film. *Am J Physics* 44 (9):813-827.

Anson, R. S. 1975. *They've killed the President. The search for the murderers of John F. Kennedy.* New York:Bantam.

Armed Forces Institute of Pathology 1960. *Autopsy manual.* Washington, D.C.: Departments of the Army, the Navy, and the Air Force.

Askins 1969. The 6.5 has a lot going for it. *Guns* 15 (9-6):22 June.

Bishop, J. 1969. *The day Kennedy was shot.* New York:Bantam.

Blumenthal, S. and H. Yazijian, eds. 1976. *Government by gunplay. Assassination conspiracy theories from Dallas to today.* New York:New American Library.

Carnes, W. H., R. S. Fisher, R. H. Morgan, and A. Moritz 1968. *Panel review of photographs, x-ray films, documents and other evidence pertaining to the fatal wounding of President John F. Kennedy on November 22, 1963, in Dallas, Texas.* Washington, D. C.:National Archives.

Ceccaldi, P. F. 1962. The examination of fire arms and ammunition. In *Methods of forensic science,* ed. F. Lundquist, pp. 593-637. New York:Interscience.

Clemedson, C. J., B. Falconer, L. Frankenberg, A. Jönsson, and J. Wennerstrand 1973. Head injuries caused by small-calibre, high velocity bullets. *Z Rechtsmed* 73:103-114.

Clinch, N. G. 1973. *The Kennedy neurosis.* New York:G&D.

Cooper, P. 1973. *The medical detectives.* New York:McKay.

Curran, W. J. and E. D. Shapiro, 1970. *Law, medicine, and forensic science,* 2nd ed., pp. 202-216. Boston:Little, Brown.

Current Medicine for Attorneys 1965. The Warren Report. How to murder the medical evidence. *Current Medicine for Attorneys* 12 (50):1-12.

Eisenberg, M. A. 1964. *Memorandum for the record. Subject: Conference of April 21, 1964, to determine which frames in the Zapruder movies show the impact of the first and second bullets.* Commission Administrative File. Washington, D. C.:National Archives.

Encyclopaedia Britannica 1964. *Book of the year for 1964,* p. 628. Chicago:William Benton, Publisher.

Facts on File 1963. November 21-27, 1963. *Facts on File from the World News Digest* 23 (1204):409.

Facts on File 1974. *Facts on File from the World News Digest* 34 (1749):

398E3.

Finck, P. S. 1966. *Missile wounds. Syllabus. M14865.* Washington, D.C.: American Registry of Pathology.

Fox, S. 1965. *The unanswered questions about President Kennedy's assassination.* New York:Award. Univ Pub & Dist.

Garrison, J. 1970. *A heritage of stone.* New York:Berkley Pub.

Gebelein, H. J. 1965. Letter to Mr. Stewart Galanor, 390 Greystone Avenue, Riverdale, New York, 10463, from Olin Mathieson Chemical Corporation. In *Rush to judgement,* ed. M. Lane, p. 411. Chicago:HR&W.

Gee, D. J. 1968. *Lecture notes on forensic medicine.* Oxford:Blackwell.

Gun Digest 1975. *1975 yearbook.* Northfield, Illinois, Digest Books.

Guy, R. D. and B. D. Pate 1973. Studies of the trace element content of bullet lead and jacket material. *J Forensic Sci* 18 (2):87-92.

Houts, M. 1967. The Warren Commission botched the Kennedy autopsy. Warren Commission one-bullet theory exploded. *Argosy* July 1967:21-22.

Humes, J. J., J. T. Boswell, J. H. Ebersole, and J. T. Stringer 1966. *Report of inspection by naval medical staff on November 1, 1966, at National Archives of x-rays and photographs of autopsy of President John F. Kennedy.*

Jacobs, N. 1967. Letter to the editor. *Ramparts* January, 1967. vol. 5 no. 7:6-7.

Lane, M. 1966. *Rush to judgement.* With an introduction by Hugh Trevor-Roper. New York:HR&W.

L'Etang, H. 1970. *The pathology of leadership.* New York:Hawthorn.

Lewis, A. 1964. Panel to reject theories of plot in Kennedy death. *New York Times,* p. 1. 1 June 1964.

Liddle, G. W. 1975. Addison's disease. In *Textbook of medicine,* 14th ed., eds. P. B. Beeson and W. McDermott, vol. 2, pp. 1736-1739. Philadelphia:Saunders.

Lockhart, R. D., G. F. Hamilton, F. W. Fyfe 1972. *Anatomy of the human body.* Philadelphia:Lippincott.

Lukash, L. I. 1974. Standards for the medical-legal investigation of death. *Tulane Medicine* 6-7 (2-3):4-5.

Marshall, E. 1975. The aftermath. *The New Republic* 173 (13):48-51.

Meagher, S. 1966. *Subject index to the Warren Report and Hearings and Exhibits.* New York:Scarecrow.

Meagher, S. 1976. *Accessories after the fact. The Warren Commission, the authorities, and the Report.* New York:Vin. Random.

Meunier, R. F. 1976. *Shadows of a doubt.* Hicksville, New York:Exposition.

Model, R. P. and R. J. Groden 1976. *JFK: The case for conspiracy.* New York:Manor Book.

Moenssens, A. A., R. E. Moses, and F. E. Inbau 1973. *Scientific evidence in criminal cases.* Mineola, New York:Foundation Press, Inc.

Morrow, R. D. 1976. *Betrayal.* Chicago:Regnery.

National Archives. *Warren Commission File No. 5*, p. 117. Washington, D.C.

NBC Log 1963. *22 November 1963*. Page 8.

The New Republic 1975. The ghost will not rest. *The New Republic* 1973 (13):7-8.

The New Republic 1975. The documents. *The New Republic* 1973 (13):12-48.

New York Times, 6 December 1963 p. 1. Warren inquiry in assassination begins its work.

New York Times, 26 January 1964 p. 58. J. Langguth: Twelve perplexing questions about Kennedy assassination examined.

New York Times, 8 December 1966 p. 40. P. Kihss: Critic of Warren Commission disputes film timing of assassination shots.

New York Times, 6 January 1967 p. 1. Rules for x-rays of Kennedy given.

New York Times, 6 January 1968, p. 15. The letter on Kennedy autopsy photos.

Newcomb, F. T. and P. Adams 1974. *Murder from within*, copy number 94. Santa Barbara, California:Published by the authors.

Newcomb, F. T. and P. Adams 1974. *Did someone alter the medical evidence?* *Skeptic* Special Issue Number 9:25-27, 61.

Nichols, J. 1973. Assassination of President Kennedy. *Practitioner* 211:625-633.

Noyes, P. 1973. *Legacy of doubt*. New York:Pinnacle Books.

O'Connor, J. 1949. *The rifle book*, p. 62. New York:Knopf.

Olson, D. and R. F. Turner 1971. Photographic evidence and the assassination of President John F. Kennedy. *J Forensic Sci* 16 (4):399-419.

O'Neill, F. X. and J. W. Sibert 1963. *Autopsy of body of President John Fitzgerald Kennedy*. Federal Bureau of Investigation File Number 89-30, 11/26/63. Commission Document Number 7. DL100-10461/CV.

Philadelphia Sunday Bulletin 1963. 24 November 1963.

President's Commission on the Assassination of President John F. Kennedy 1964. *Report*. Washington, D.C.:U.S. Government Printing Office.

Prouty, L. F. 1973. *The secret team*. Englewood Cliffs, New Jersey:P-H.

Rockefeller, N. 1975. *Report to the President by the Commission on CIA Activities within the United States*. New York:Manor Book.

Scott, P. D., P. L. Hoch, and R. Stetler eds. 1976. *The assassinations. Dallas and beyond*. New York:Vin. Random.

Sellier, K. 1971. Ueber Geschossablenkung und Geschossdeformation. *Z Rechtsmed* 69:217-251.

Smith, J. E. 1969. *Small arms of the world*, 9th rev. ed. Harrisburg:Stackpole.

Spitz, W. U. and R. S. Fisher eds. 1973. *Medicolegal investigation of death*. Springfield:Thomas.

State of Louisiana v. Clay Shaw 1969. Testimony of Pierre A. Finck, February 25, 1969.

Szulc, T. 1975. The Warren Commission in its own words. *The New Republic* 173 (13):9-12.

Tamaska, L. 1964. Kritische Bemerken zu Frage der

Geschosskaliberbestimmung aus dem Durchmesser der Einschussöffnungen der Knochen. *Zacchia* 27:158-170.

Taylor, H. L. 1974. The general pathologist and the medicolegal autopsy. *Arch Pathol* 98:426-429.

Texas Journal of Medicine 1964. Three patients at Parkland. *Texas J Med* 60:61-74.

Thompson, J. 1976. *Six second in Dallas.* New York:Berkley Medallion Book.

Thorwald, J. 1965. *The century of the detective.* New York:Harcourt, Brace and World.

United Press International 1964. *Four days. The historical record of the death of President Kennedy.* New York:Am Heritage.

Washington Post 1963. 18 December 1963.

Washington Post 1966. 29 May 1966.

Wecht, C. H. 1966. A critique of the medical aspects of the investigation into the assassination of President Kennedy. *J Forensic Sci* 11:300-316.

Wecht, C. H. 1974. JFK assassination. A prolonged and willful coverup. *Modern Medicine.*

Wecht, C. H. and R. P. Smith 1974. Medical evidence in the assassination of President John F. Kennedy. In *Legal medicine annual,* ed. C. H. Wecht, pp. 69-98. New York:Appleton.

Weisberg, H. 1965. *Whitewash. The report on the Warren Report.* New York:Dell Book.

Wilber, C. G. 1974. *Forensic biology for the law enforcement officer.* Springfield:Thomas.

Wilber, C. G. 1977. *Ballistic science for the law enforcement officer.* Springfield:Thomas.

Wrone, D. R. 1972. The assassination of John Fitzgerald Kennedy. *Wisconsin Magazine of History* 56:21-36.

Young, B. C. and C. J. Stahl 1966. *Gunshot wounds. Syllabus. L12066.* Washington, D.C.: American Registry of Pathology.

INDEX

311